Medicinal Plants
of North America

Help Us Keep This Guide Up to Date

Every effort has been made by the author and editors to make this guide as accurate and useful as possible.

We would love to hear from you concerning your experiences with this guide and how you feel it could be improved and kept up to date. While we may not be able to respond to all comments and suggestions, we'll take them to heart, and we'll also make certain to share them with the author. Please send your comments and suggestions to the following address:

The Globe Pequot Press
Reader Response/Editorial Department
P.O. Box 480
Guilford, CT 06437

Or you may e-mail us at:

editorial@globepequot.com

Thanks for your input, and happy hunting!

MEDICINAL PLANTS OF NORTH AMERICA

A Field Guide

Jim Meuninck

FALCONGUIDES ®

GUILFORD, CONNECTICUT
HELENA, MONTANA
AN IMPRINT OF THE GLOBE PEQUOT PRESS

FALCONGUIDES®

Text design by Mary Ballachino
Photo credits: Betty Combs p. 48; Stan Combs p. 147; Gerald O. Dudley, Ph.D., pp. 148-49; Russ Schneider pp. 126, 134. All other photographs by Jim Meuninck

Library of Congress Cataloging-in-Publication Data

Meuninck, Jim, 1942-
    Medicinal plants of North America : a field guide / Jim Meuninck. — 1st ed.
        p. cm.
    Includes bibliographical references and index.
    ISBN-13: 978-0-7627-4298-1
    1. Medicinal plants—North America—Identification. I. Title.
    QK110.M48 2008
    581.6′34097—dc22

                                                                                2007030688

Printed in China
10 9 8 7 6 5 4 3 2 1

To buy books in quantity for corporate use
or incentives, call **(800) 962–0973**
or e-mail **premiums@GlobePequot.com.**

The health information expressed in this book is based solely on the personal experience of the author and is not intended as a medical manual. The information should not be used for diagnosis or treatment, or as a substitute for professional medical care. The identification, selection, and processing of any wild plant for use as food or medicine requires reasonable care and attention to details since, as indicated in the text, certain parts are wholly unsuitable for use and in some instances are toxic. The author and publisher urge you to consult with your health-care provider prior to using any wild plant as food or medicine.

The natural world is not something alien and wild. It is not an enemy or outside force that must be sub-dued and dominated.

—JAMAKE HIGHWATER, *THE PRIMAL MIND*

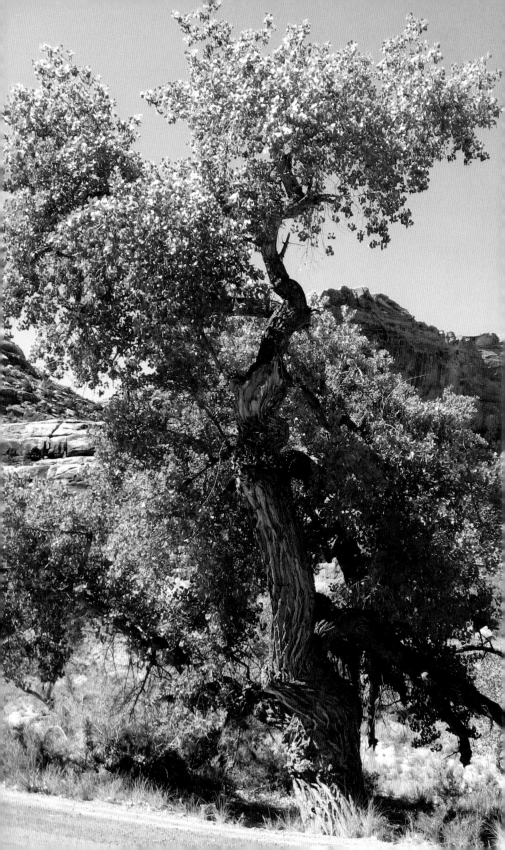

Contents

Left: Cottonwood in the Southwest

Chapter 2: Medicinal Herbs of Eastern Forested Areas | 51

Chapter 3: Woody Plants of Eastern Forests, Yards, Meadows, and Roadsides | 69

Preface

First the word, then the plant, lastly the knife.

—AESCULAPIUS 1200 B.C.

In 1985, after I had been making educational films for ten years, my government grants evaporated and I found myself in an unemployment line fidgeting with my keys. A $99 check was my reward for surviving another week. I took the money, rented a broadcast video camera, left home for ten weeks, and began an odyssey: filming edible and medicinal wild plants. I plodded through forests, forded streams, climbed mountains, and mucked through swamps, grabbing short clips of useful wildflowers (and they are all useful). When it was over, I had a film, still had my family, and had accrued a great deal of debt. Debt to my wife, Jill, and daughter, Rebecca; debt to Dr. Jim Duke, who coauthored my first video; and debt to Steven Foster, whose kind reviews induced the Boy Scouts of America and Outdoor Life Book Club to distribute the program. With the proceeds from sales, I built a production studio, and now—fourteen videos and three books later—I continue to discover the surprising benefits of our native flora.

Although the dampness has dried behind my ears, the echoes of experts still reverberate. These echoes remind me that all medicinal plant compendiums are collaborations with those who went before. So I thank them all: Native Americans, American pioneers, and the thousands of herbalists prior and the thousands after. Discovering and sharing their knowledge is what this book is about, so I humbly submit their wisdom with a few fresh ideas of my own.

The production of this book was made possible with the help of Paula Brisco, who kept the train from derailing; Shelley Wolf, who nurtured the engine along with patience and sound advice; and Mary Ballachino, who gave it all a place to go. Thank you to the American Botanical Council, who provided a push to put me over the hill, and thanks to Candace Corson, MD, whose insight and wisdom made this a more useful and more accurate guide.

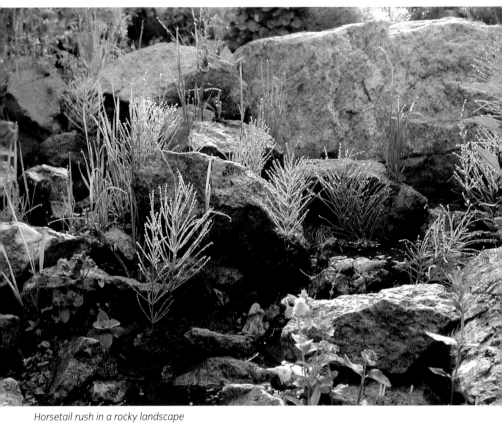

Horsetail rush in a rocky landscape

Introduction: What Are Medicinal Plants?

The onset of agriculture brought with it a surge of infections, a decline in the overall quality of nutrition, and reduction in the average length of life.

—COHEN ET AL., PALEOPATHOLOGY AT THE ORIGINS OF AGRICULTURE

Medicinal plants and wild plant foods provide chemicals your body needs to maintain optimum health. Your organ systems want to be whole and healthy, and medicinal plants can induce body functions in the direction they need to go. Wild plants cleanse and strengthen body tissues and organ systems. They energize your brain, improve your diet, nourish and cleanse your organ systems, provide physical energy, strengthen immunity, and provide first-line defense against the degenerative diseases of aging. With the selective use of plants you can lower blood cholesterol levels, lower blood pressure, prevent strokes, and help prevent cancer. Bear in mind that plants are less a cure for disease than a *preventive*. The body wants to heal, and herbs help.

This book is a field guide, not a prescription for medicinal plants. Medicinal plants should only be used with the guidance and oversight of a professional, holistic health-care practitioner. Pregnant and lactating women should never use wild plants as therapy without professional supervision. Keep in mind that each human being is unique and that each person's reaction to chemicals from wild plants varies: *What is my food may be your poison*. Take personal responsibility for your health, get advice from experts, feed your intellect, and step lively and wisely through life.

Before going afield, let's discover how plants have helped the human species endure and proliferate.

You Are Plants with Wheels

You either eat plants or eat animals that eat plants; therefore, your body's chemistry is made from plant chemistry. In effect, you are a plant with wheels. Plants contain all the essential and nonessential nutrients and chemicals you need. The vegetables, roots, and fruits that you eat and the herbs you sprinkle over food are full of health-protecting chemicals that are antiviral, antibacterial, antiasthmatic, anti-inflammatory, and antifungal.

Where do plants get this power? Consider this: A typical tomato produces more than 10,000 unique physiologically active compounds. Many of these chemicals are used by the plant to germinate, grow, flower, and propagate. But thousands of others have more mysterious uses. What are they for? Unlike you, a plant doesn't have legs; it cannot run and hide from its enemies. It is firmly stuck in the earth, unable to escape predators that would destroy or devour it. To survive plants produce thousands of chemicals, called secondary metabolites, that fend off or kill viruses, bacteria, nematodes, and myriad other creatures that would do them harm. When you eat plants these potent chemicals are taken into your body and utilized. In effect many ingested plant chemicals protect you by staving off enemies that might do you harm.

That's how medicinal plants work: They induce, expel, stimulate, organize, warm, rebuild, and protect. This is not new information. For thousands of years plants have been humankind's primary medicine. They have also been used to flavor and preserve food. Before refrigeration was invented, our ancestors sprinkled combinations of salt and herbs over foods as preservatives to slow degradation and provide flavors and aromas that masked the foul taste and funky odor of rancid food. At the same time the herbal preservatives packed a bonus dose of health-protecting chemistry.

These combinations of indigenous medicinal herbs give a particular ethnic food its characteristic flavor and have come to be known as cultural flavor principles. Curry is a traditional example of a cultural flavor principle that preserves food and provides health benefits. Research suggests that cultural flavor principles play a key role in protecting health and increasing longevity. Flavor principles help explain why the Japanese, Greeks, and Italians live longer than Americans. When you learn to prepare foods with cultural flavor principles that contain medicinal plants, you reap better health and a longer life.

Chemical Families

There are several important families of plant chemicals: polysaccharides, simple sugars, proteins, oils, bioflavonoids, sterols, acids, and alkaloids. These chemical families and their members are composed of thousands of physiologically active compounds. Dr. Jim Duke, former chief of germplasm at the U.S. Department of Agriculture (USDA), has compiled a huge database of plants and their physiologically active chemicals. Visit his Web site (www.ars-grin.gov/duke) to discover which plants have what chemicals and how those chemicals effect human physiology.

You will soon learn that many plants are used in similar ways—that literally hundreds of plants treat diarrhea; that all plants contain cancer-fighting antioxidants (some more, some less); that all roots store immune-stimulating polysaccharides; that you have a broad choice of anti-inflammatory plant foods; and that gas-relieving digestives come in

Herbal Preparations Defined

Modern technology provides superior ways of distilling, extracting, purifying, and standardizing herbal extracts that are beyond the scope of this book (see appendixes C and D for additional resources). But let us define some terms in this book.

Tea (also known as infusion or tisane) is prepared by pouring hot water (just off the boil) over fresh or dried herbs. Typically the soft parts (leaves and flowering parts) of the plant are infused. *Examples:* green teas, black teas, herbal teas. *Amount:* One teaspoon dried herb to 1 cup of water; 4 teaspoons of fresh herb to 1 cup of water.

Decoction: A liquid made by simmering or boiling herbs in water. Decoctions pull water-soluble chemistry from the hard parts of the plant: the stems, seeds, bark, and roots. *Example:* Garlic soup. *Amount:* One teaspoon dried herb to 1 cup of water; 4 teaspoons fresh herb to 1 cup of water.

Percolation is like making coffee: Water or alcohol is dripped through a damp mass of powdered herb. *Example:* Dripping hot water or alcohol through cayenne powder. Put a drop to your lips. . . . Zowee! *Amount:* One hundred milliliters of liquid through 10 grams dried herb; repeat the process over and over to increase concentration.

Tinctures: Chopping and blending an herb in alcohol. Other chemicals can be used, such as apple cider vinegar or glycerin. The maceration (blending) can be accomplished in a blender. *Example:* Blend 100 proof alcohol (Everclear) with fresh echinacea flowers. Cut the whole flowers in small pieces, place in a blender, cover with Everclear and macerate. Let the maceration rest in the refrigerator for four hours, then strain and bottle. *Amount:* When making a tincture with a dry herb, typically a 1:5 ratio is used—that is, 1 ounce of the dried herb is macerated and blended with 5 ounces of 50% (100 proof) alcohol. With fresh herbs a 1:2 ration is often used—1 gram to every cubic centimeter of 50% (100 proof) alcohol.

Fomentation: Prepare a decoction or infusion of herbs (see above), then dip a cotton cloth into the preparation and wrap the warm wet cotton cloth around an injury. *Example:* Dipping a cloth in a mild cayenne extraction and applying it to an arthritic joint. (*Note:* This application will redden the skin and may irritate.) *Amount:* Enough to cover area to be treated.

Poultice: Pound and macerate fresh herbs and apply the moist herb mass directly over a body part. *Example:* Putting a warm, wet, and pounded mass of plantain over a pus-filled wound. *Amount:* Large enough amount to cover area to be treated.

Powders are prepared by drying and finely grinding the herb, then loading the powder into a 00 capsule. *Example:* Many over-the-counter dried herbs are sold in capsules. *Amount:* Typically one 500- to 1,000-milligram capsule.

Oils and salves are prepared with dried or fresh herbs. First the herb is cooked in oil to extract the active principle, then the oil is thickened or hardened with beeswax. *Example:* The aerial parts (flowers, leaves, and stems) of yarrow are simmered in oil and then blended with warm beeswax. The blend is cooled, and the resulting salve is applied as a wound treatment. *Amount:* With yarrow I lightly pack a pan with fresh leaves and flowers and cover with olive oil or lard (studies suggest lard is better absorbed through human skin than plant oils).

many shapes, colors, and flavors. Once aware of this overlap, you should strive to make *food* your medicine—that is, eat *edible* plants that have proven medicinal value. And play it safe: Avoid medicinal plants that are not considered safe food.

Here's how I use medicinal plants as food: To improve digestion and assimilation of meals, I eat safe bitter herbs in my salads. I snip dandelion leaves, chop them small, and throw them in a bowl with some mesclun mix (lettuce, arugula, a bit of chopped chicory leaves) and maybe some fresh basil, oregano, and purslane. Now I have a salad with slightly bitter, edible medicinal herbs that streamline digestion and assimilation, provide me with pain-relieving anti-inflammation chemistry, and offer cancer-fighting antioxidants.

Here's another scenario: Let's say your child comes home from school with a cold—you don't want to catch that. So place a thin slice of raw sweet potato on a piece of bread. Pull a burdock root from your yard and shred that over the sweet potato. Maybe grate just a little raw horseradish root on top. Then, if available, plug in a couple of thin slices of raw Jerusalem artichoke root. Slather a second piece of bread with pesto, flip on a few dill pickle slices, cover with lettuce, and slip in some ham, beef, or whatever you like. Voilà—you have an infection-fighting sandwich. Finish the meal with ten drops of echinacea and that should hammer the cold before it takes hold. The raw medicinal plant roots provide immune-stimulating polysaccharides, and the echinacea has a sterling history of fighting acute infections, especially when the infection is caught early.

Herbal teas are another example of herbs as food. Teas are used in traditional medicine to stimulate and cleanse organ systems. They can protect you from infection, open your sinuses, quell your cough, fight heart disease, prevent cancer, move your bowels, and relax your mind. In rural India and many other places around the world, foul drinking water is boiled and infused with aromatic herbs to mask the taste and disguise the water's odor. Herbal teas can also make you vomit, give you diarrhea, induce hallucinations, and cause death. This book will explain which herbs are beneficial and which ones are dangerous.

In fact, herbs are used in many health-affirming ways, including:

- **Managing blood pressure and cholesterol.** Eating more plant foods and using less salt help manage blood pressure. Green plant foods and herbs are diuretics. For example, research showed that capsicum, derived from cayenne and jalapeño peppers, increases blood flow, lowering both blood pressure and cholesterol.

  Numerous studies have shown the benefits of garlic. It balances cholesterol levels in the blood by lowering serum cholesterol and raising HDL cholesterol. Garlic is also anticlotting, reducing plaque formation in blood vessels.

  Other herbs found in America such as ginseng, aloe vera, dandelion, black cohosh, yellow dock, burdock, echinacea, and red clover blossoms all have blood-pressure-lowering and cholesterol-lowering chemistry.

- **Treating cancer.** Mayapple contains podophyllotoxin. A synthetic analog of podophyllotoxin is used to treat small-cell lung cancer and testicular cancer. Ellagic acid from the seeds of berries, specifically raspberries, has proven useful as an adjuvant nutritional therapy for cancer patients. Flaxseed oil is being studied as a cancer therapy. Traditional treatments that are scientifically unproven, like the Essiac formula, are discussed in the text. Vegetables, fruits, nuts, and herbs provide substantial amounts of cancer-fighting antioxidants.

- **Treating arthritis.** Compound P from cayenne is used to quell pain and improve circulation to arthritic joints. Stinging nettle is often used in Mexico to alleviate severe arthritic pain. The nettle is slapped over the joint as a counterirritant, and the resulting sting and inflammation is said to bring relief. Other North American medicinal plants used as adjuvant nutritional therapy for arthritis include lime juice, white willow, wild strawberry, spruce, flaxseed oil, raw green wild plants, almonds, walnuts, and pine nuts.

- **Influencing sexual drive.** Chemicals from certain herbs may affect sexual desire and sexual function in humans. Traditionally American ginseng, saw palmetto, marijuana, passionflower, lady's slipper, and California poppy have been used to affect libido.

How to Use This Book

This field guide offers a unique identification system: It moves the user from the simple and familiar plants to the rare and complex. It builds from a solid foundation of basic

Germany's Commission E

Throughout this guide you'll find references to Commission E, Germany's official government agency specifically focused on herbs. In 1978 the Bundesgesundheitsamt (a federal health agency similar to the U.S. Food and Drug Administration) organized the commission to evaluate the safety and efficacy of medicinal herbs. The commission's broad range of interdisciplinary experience and expertise is unique in the world: Its twenty-four members include physicians, pharmacists, pharmacologists, toxicologists, representatives of the pharmaceutical industry, and laypeople.

The Commission E monographs consist of more than 300 articles on herbal preparations that serve as the basis for the use of these plant drugs within the German health-care system. Monographs include the name of the herb, its constituents, indications for use, contraindications, side effects, interactions with other drugs, and dosage. The complete text of the Commission E monographs was translated and published in English in 1998 by the Austin, Texas–based American Botanical Council. For more information visit the council's Web site at www.herbalgram.org.

information and takes the forager as far as he or she wants to go. The goal is to help the reader identify plants that have been used as medicine for thousands of years.

Each entry begins with a description—a summary of the plant's physical characteristics to aid in plant identification, followed by an explanation of the location, the part of the country where the plant grows.

We then discuss the plant's role past and present as food, its traditional medicinal uses (including how it was used by American Indians and by American pioneers), and its modern medicinal uses.

Throughout this book you will learn which herbs are beneficial and which ones are dangerous. The caution sections give details about plants' dangerous characteristics or uses.

In the notes I share experiences, skills, gardening tips, recipes, and bits of humor gleaned from my forty-plus years of using herbs.

The wildlife/veterinary uses section presents unique observations and useful experiences relevant to animal lovers and naturalists.

The plant entries provide a wealth of supplemental Web sites, books, and research references. You'll find other useful information and resources in this guide's appendixes.

Now take the first step toward a longer, healthier, more productive life: Sit down and read this book, then hike afield and discover health-improving herbs that grow as near as your own backyard.

CHAPTER 1

Medicinal Plants of Yards, Prairies, Roadsides, and Meadows

> When we destroy a people's experience, they
> become destructive.
>
> —R. D. LAING

These common plants are often found growing in yards, along roadsides, and in open areas. They are easily transplanted to your garden.

Dandelion
Taraxacum officinale G.H. Weber
ex Wiggers

Description: Perennial weed with a basal whorl of toothed leaves. Yellow composite flower with numerous rays born on 6- to 10-inch flower stem. Torn leaf or flower stem exudes white-colored latex.

Location: Worldwide, temperate regions. Common yard bounty.

Food: A vitamin- and mineral-rich salad green. Tear it into small pieces (leave out the tough veins) for salad and mix with thyme, fennel, nasturtiums, and salad greens. Thyme and fennel balance the dandelion's bitterness. Make a mineral-rich tea from dandelion roots and leaves. Gently simmer chopped fresh roots for a stomach bitters; the bitter brew will stimulate the flow of gastric acid and bile, improving digestion and assimilation. Cook fresh leaves gathered early in the season with olive oil, bacon, and lemon

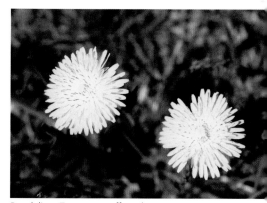

Dandelion, *Taraxacum officinale*

juice. As the season progresses, dandelion leaves become more bitter: Pour copious amount of water on the late-summer plants so that the morning harvest will be sweeter. Even when bitter, the leaves are a healthy addition to stir-fries. Try dandelion with tofu. Cook the leaves in oyster oil with cayenne, garlic, and beef strips.

Traditional uses: The root decoction is a liver-cleansing tonic that aids digestion and helps cleanse the blood. It is also diuretic and is traditionally used to treat premenstrual syndrome (PMS). It has a mild laxative effect and may relieve inflammation and congestion of the gall-bladder and liver. Native Americans applied a poultice of steamed dandelion leaves to treat stomachaches. Greens were considered a tonic blood purifier. The root decoction was imbibed to increase lactation and was used as mild laxative and for dyspepsia.

Modern uses: Commission E–approved for treating dyspeptic complaints, urinary infections, liver and gallbladder com-plaints, and appetite loss. Root extract may lower cholesterol and blood pres-sure (hypotensive). Dandelion is one of the most potent diuretics. Its perform-ance in animal studies is equal to the pre-scription drug furosemide. Dandelions are a stimulating tonic and mild laxative with blood-glucose-regulating capacity. The bitter taste of dandelion is an appetite stimulant and stimulates the entire digestive system (cholagogue), improving appetite, and may be helpful treating anorexia. It raises hydrochloric acid secretion in the stomach, improving calcium breakdown and absorption, and it also spurs bile production.

Dandelion and other bitter high-fiber greens can theoretically lower cholesterol in three ways: 1) Eating the leaves stimu-lates the secretion of bile, requiring more production of bile from cholesterol. 2) Fiber in the plants locks up bile in the digestive tract, arresting cholesterol breakdown and emulsification, thus pre-venting cholesterol absorption. 3) Fiber

removes bile from the body, causing the liver to convert more cholesterol into bile. These factors help prevent athero-sclerosis, reduce stroke, and lower blood pressure.

Notes: Eight plants grown under lights or in a window provide ample edible leaves for two people. We eat dandelion greens and make root tea year-round. Bring plants indoors for the winter. Late-season bitter leaves can be chopped and added to salads. Flower petals may be sprinkled over salads, rice dishes, and vegetable dishes.

Wildlife/veterinary uses: Goldfinches eat the seeds, which is another great rea-son to grow this plant in your lawn. Dried dandelion root and dandelion tea are an integral constituent of my pigeon racing formulas. A fertility-improving herbal sup-plement for horses called Fertility Boost contains dandelion. Another horse prod-uct uses dandelion as part of a formula for improving, strengthening, and reliev-ing problems with a horse's feet. Brain Cool, a horse product, is combined with many herbs as a supplement for working animals.

Plantain
Plantago lanceolata L.; *P. major* L.; *P. maritima* L.

Description: Several varieties are found across the United States. Leaves in a basal whorl. Flower stem height may reach 8 to 10 inches. The difference is in the leaves. *P. major* leaves are broad, ovate. *P. lanceolata* leaves are narrow and lance shaped. *P. maritima* leaves are

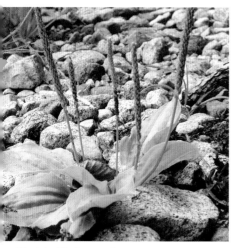

Plantain, *Plantago major*

narrower, almost linear; this species is found along the Pacific coast, often submerged during high tide. The green flowers of all three species are born on terminal spikes.

Location: Nationwide. Open ground, wasteland, edges of fields and roads, lawns. *P. maritima* is found in the upper tidal zone.

Food: In the spring I pluck whole leaves from my garden and yard and chop them into salads or sauté them with wild leeks, nettles, and watercress. Tear out the tough midleaf vein (rib) from summer and autumn leaves before adding them to salads.

Traditional uses: The flowering heads may be stripped off by running the stem between thumb and forefinger. Add the flower heads to hot water to form a mucilaginous drink for treating constipation. A few folks believe that this plant, when crushed and applied to the skin, is a good antidote or treatment for poison

ivy. Native Americans chewed the leaves to produce an antiseptic and immune-stimulating poultice for wounds, scrapes, cuts, and bruises. The poultice stops blood flow (styptic). You can use plantain the same way today—simply chew the plantain leaf and fix it in place over the wound. Defensin, a chemical in our mouth, is antibiotic and stimulates the immune system. Digestive enzymes in our saliva are also weakly antimicrobial. Plantain lotions and ointments are used to treat hemorrhoids, skin fistulae, and ulcers. The tea is a diuretic, decongestant, and expectorant and may be helpful in treating diarrhea, dysentery, irritable bowel syndrome, laryngitis, and urinary tract bleeding. Acubin from plantain increases uric acid excretion by kidneys and may be helpful in treating gout.

Modern uses: Commission E reports that *P. lanceolata* extract from the fresh plant may fight colds (4 grams of herb to 1 cup boiling water), may alleviate symptoms of bronchitis and cough, and may reduce fever. It is approved for treating inflammation of the pharynx and mouth and for skin inflammations. Typically, a dose is 3 to 6 grams of the fresh whole herb (aerial parts when in bloom); add all to 1 cup of water just off the boil. Let it cool, strain away plant material, then drink. This beverage may be taken three or four times a day. The tea of the fresh leaves is also used to treat respiratory tract infections and is considered antibacterial.

Notes: Plantago seeds of India and Africa are dried and used as a bulking laxative. *P. ovata* is a constituent of Metamucil.

Wildlife/veterinary uses: *P. major* is a favored food of the eastern box turtle. Tough leaf veins can be stripped and in an emergency used as fish line, even used as suture material for saving a hunting dog bitten by a bear. Psyllium seed is used in training mixes and wound-treatment formulas for horses.

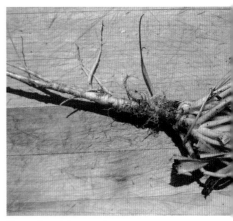

Queen Anne's lace root

Queen Anne's Lace, Wild Carrot

Daucus carota L.

Description: Biennial to 3 feet in height. First-year plant prostrate and spreading; featherlike leaves, deeply cut, inconspicuous in deep weeds. Torn leaf has odor of carrot. Second-year plant bears white florets in round umbels on 3- to 4-foot stems. Carrot-scented flowers.

Location: Nationwide. Meadows, waste ground, roadsides, vacant lots.

Food: Wild carrot, or Queen Anne's lace, is widely available. We use the florets in salads to get a healthy dose of bioflavonoids that may improve distal circulation to the brain and the extremities and may improve heart function. Seeds are used for flavoring. The first year's raw root is eaten in salads, juiced, or cooked as a vegetable. The second-year root may be eaten but is woody and only flavors the food it is cooked with. Outer root flesh may be nibbled off the woody center after it has been softened by cooking.

CAUTION: Many members of this family (Apiaceae) are delicious (lovage, carrot, fennel, and others). But a few, like cow parsnip, may cause a photoallergic reaction when handled. Others like poison hemlock and water hemlock are fatally toxic. One way to be certain you have carrot and not a toxic variety is to plant your own carrots, leave a few in the ground after the first year, and the second-year growth will bear the characteristic umbel of blooms.

Traditional uses: Pioneers used the oil in skin creams as an antiwrinkle agent, a practice that continues today. The whole

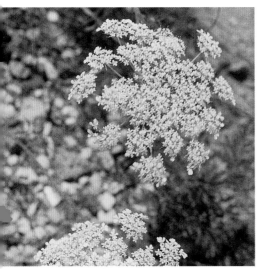

Queen Anne's lace, *Daucus carota*

plant was infused and used to wash wounds and sores and as a hair rinse. Flowers were infused and the resulting drink was consumed to treat diabetes. Roots were decocted and used as a wash and also as a tonic to balance blood chemistry, treat acne, and as a diuretic to increase urination. Root decoction is said to be an appetite stimulant. Micmac First Peoples used the leaves to purge bowels.

Modern uses: Carrot roots and leaves contain carotenoids, which are helpful in preventing cancer. Tea of the whole plant and seeds is used to treat urinary problems, such as cystitis or stones. Seeds are antiflatulent. Seed and root are used to treat edema. Oil of seed is an ingredient in many commercial skin products. Seeds are stimulating. The carotenoid content of the root may preserve eyesight and help prevent cancer. Whole, unjuiced carrots may help lower blood sugar (antidiabetic). Eating carrots may help reduce symptoms of gout by eliminating uric acid.

Notes: Let garden carrots go to seed by not pulling the first year's roots. Collect second-year seeds for seasoning and medicinal uses. Wild carrot root may be cooked with other wild foods to add carrotlike flavor, but the core of the second-year root is tough and woody. A soft layer of edible tissue covers the woody core; scrape and peel this outer tissue from the core and eat.

Wildlife/veterinary uses: Carrot roots and leaves are fodder for chickens, pigs, exotic birds, and ungulates (animals with hooves).

Poisonous Look-alikes

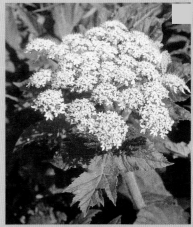
Cow parsnip, *Heracleum maximum*

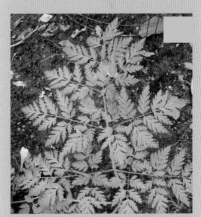
Poison hemlock, *Conium maculatum*

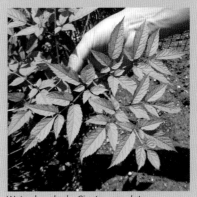
Water hemlock, *Cicuta maculata*

Goldenrod
Solidago canadensis L.

Description: Perennial, with numerous species that grow to 3 feet in height. *S. canadensis* is the most common eastern species, with a smooth stem at the base; its stem is hairy just below flower branches. Sharp-toothed leaves plentiful, lance shaped, with three veins. Golden flowers line up atop stem in a broad, branched spire or triangular-shaped cluster (panicle). Plant found most often in colonies. Flowers July to September.

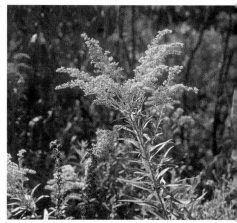

Goldenrod, *Solidago canadensis*

Location: Nationwide. Fields, meadows, roadsides, railroad right-of-ways, vacant lots, edges of fields.

Food: Seeds, shoots, and leaves are edible although bitter. Flowers can be made into a mild tea or used as a garnish on salads and other cold or hot dishes.

Traditional uses: Goldenrod is not the weed that causes autumn allergies—that's ragweed. Informants say that goldenrod tea made of fresh or dried flowers may protect a person from allergens (hypoallergenic). Dried leaves and flowers were applied to wounds to stop bleeding (styptic). Traditional herbalists and pioneers used the tea to ward off acute infections like colds, flu, and bronchitis, as it induces the production of mucus. Whole-plant tea is a kidney tonic (diuretic).

Modern uses: Commission E–approved for kidney and bladder stones as well as urinary tract infections. Plants gathered when in flower and then dried are used in Europe as a relaxant (spasmolytic) and anti-inflammatory. The drug is 6 to 12 grams dried aerial parts in infusion. People with kidney and bladder problems should only use the herb under medical supervision.

Notes: According to the *PDR for Herbal Medicines* (third edition), the herb "has a weak potential for sensitization (can cause allergies)." Thus, use of the plant drug may cause allergic reaction. Also, the whole plant can be used as a yellow dye.

Wildlife/veterinary uses: Goldenrod nectar and pollen attract bees, butterflies, wasps, moths, flies, and other insects. Caterpillars, aphids, and other small insects eat the leaves and stems. Wasps, spiders, praying mantis, lacewings, ambush bugs, assassin bugs, beetles, and birds prey on these feasting insects. There is a goldenrod spider that inhabits the plants. Gallflies lay eggs in the stems and leaves. Insect-devouring praying mantis lay their eggs on goldenrod because of its insect-attracting power. The aerial parts infused were used to treat snakebite.

Stinging Nettle
Urtica dioica L.

Description: Erect perennial to 5 feet in height. Square, grooved stem, studded with stinging hairs. Leaves dark green, rough, heart to oval shaped, toothed. Green flowers born in leaf axils, bearing numerous green seeds. Both sexes on one plant and plants with separate sexes.

Location: Nationwide. Edges of fields, streamside, wetlands, marshy areas, fringe areas, wasteland, roadsides.

Food: Young shoots in fall (new growth) and shoots in spring are picked and steamed, sautéed, or stir-fried. One of my favorite recipes is cream of nettle soup.

Older, summer-hardened nettles may be simmered with other herbs (rosemary, celery, thyme, onions, leeks, and lovage) to make a vegetable bouillon or soup base. Discard the plant material after simmering for twenty-five minutes, then use the broth in cooking.

Traditional uses: Nettles, a mineral-rich plant food, have been used for generations to treat allergies. The infusion of the aerial parts has expectorant qualities and was used for asthma and cough. Nettle tincture is used for flu, colds, pneumonia, and bronchitis. Dried plant is styptic when applied to wounds, and naturopaths use the drug to treat internal bleeding. According to Steve Brill and

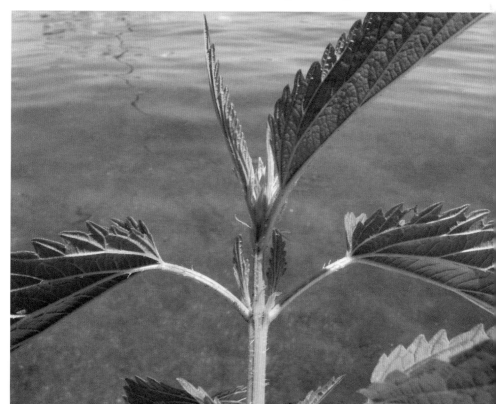

Stinging nettle, *Urtica dioica*

Evelyn Dean in their book *Identifying and Harvesting Edible and Medicinal Plants in Wild (and Not So Wild) Places,* drinking nettle tea and eating nettles may make your skin clearer and healthier and it may be therapeutic for eczema. Eating nettles may improve color, texture, gloss, and health of hair. Aerial parts were infused as a tea and used to treat urinary tract infections, kidney and bladder stones, and rheumatism. Root tincture was used for irritable bladder and prostate complaints.

In traditional Russian medicine, nettle is used to treat hepatitis. In Spanish traditional medicine, nettle leaves are prepared in infusion as a diuretic, to replenish minerals, as a hemostat, and as a purgative to remove toxins from the body. The root is believed to reduce the size of kidney stones. A decoction of the seeds is believed to prevent involuntary urination in children.

Stinging nettle is said to be helpful on arthritic joints as a counterirritant. Using nettles to thrash arthritic joints causes pain and inflammation and temporary relief of arthritic area. This approach is not recommended. Mexican truck drivers use the plant to relieve sciatica. They also drink copious amounts of tequila. I recommend if you use the nettle arthritis remedy, have the tequila ready. Scarification is another way that Native Americans treated arthritis. For details view the DVDs *Native American Medicine* and *Little Medicine* (see appendix D).

Modern uses: Commission E–approved for treating benign prostatic hyperplasia (BPH). Nettle root and saw palmetto have been combined successfully to treat prostate enlargement symptoms (Engleman et al., "Efficacy and Safety of a Combination of Sabal and Urtica Extract in Lower Urinary Tract Symptoms," *Arzneim-Forschung/Drug Research* 56, no. 3 [2006]: 2222–29). Nettle roots in Russia are tinctured for hepatitis and gallbladder inflammation. In Germany, as in the United States, nettle root extract is being researched as a treatment for prostate problems.

A randomized study of arthritis sufferers suggests that stinging nettle extract, when accompanied by a lowered dose of the anti-inflammatory drug diclofenac (used for treating arthritis), improved or enhanced the efficacy of the prescription drug (Chrubasik et al., "Evidence for Antirheumatic Effectiveness of Herb *Urticae dioicae* in Acute Arthritis: A Pilot Study," *Phytomedicine* 4, no. 2 [1997]: 105–8. Ramm et al., "Brennesselblatterextrakt Bei Arthrose und Rheumatoider Arthritis," *Therapiewoche* 28 [1996]: 3–6).

Notes: Stinging nettle grows readily in my garden. It provides minerals, vitamins, and phytochemistry that protects me and alleviates my psoriasis. We eat the herb stewed, steamed, or sautéed almost daily from April through October. Simply snip off new-growth leaves from the top of the plant, cook, and enjoy its multiple benefits. If you cannot obtain fresh nettle, then freeze-dried is your next best choice. Try rubbing out the sting of nettle with mullein leaves or the juice of spotted touch-me-not (jewelweed, *Impatiens capensis*).

Veterinarian/wildlife uses: Nettle is eaten by domestic animals and by chamois, a wild goatlike animal of the Pyrenees. Nettle is a vital ingredient in the cleansing tea I make for racing pigeons. Short-haired hunting dogs may have bad encounters with stinging nettle and wood nettle when hunting. Grazing animals will not eat live nettle but will eat it dried. Nettle juice mixed with nettle seeds is a good hair tonic for domestic animals (see www.ruralvermont.com).

Yarrow
Achillea millefolium L.

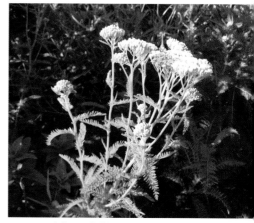

Yarrow, *Achillea millefolium*

Description: Spreading perennial to 3 or 4 feet in height. Soft, featherlike leaves. Fragrant. White flowers in flat clusters; flowers have five petal-like rays.

Location: Broadly distributed nationwide. Roadsides, fields, yards, gardens, edges of woods.

Food: Not considered a food, but see notes.

Traditional uses: Traditionally the tea made from the aerial parts (leaves and flowers) is said to increase perspiration and reduce inflammation; it is used both externally and internally. In China the tea is taken to protect against thrombosis after stroke or heart attack and is used over wounds and for hemorrhoids, inflamed eyes, nosebleeds, and ulcers. It can be combined with elderberry flowers or berries. Native Americans have infused the aerial parts of the plant to treat acute infections (colds, fever, flu), as a diuretic, to control coughing, and as a wash for bites, stings, snakebites. Root decoction was a wash for pimples. Leaves were infused and used to induce sleep, to treat poison ivy, as an antidiarrheal, to reduce

fever (febrifuge), as an astringent to treat internal and external bleeding (styptic), and to treat conditions causing bloody urine such as kidney and bladder infections. Leaves were dried, crushed, and snorted as snuff for headaches or placed in the nose to stop bleeding. Fresh or dry leaves were applied as a poultice over wounds or breast (nipple) abscesses. Leaf decoction was a hair rinse. Bella Coola peoples chewed leaves and applied them as a poultice to treat burns and boils. Leaves and flowers in decoction were used for headaches or for chest pains. Poultice of masticated flowers was applied to reduce edema. Leaves mixed with animal grease were used as a poultice on chest and back to treat bronchitis. Juice of aerial parts or decoction of aerial parts was considered a general tonic.

Modern uses: Commission E–approved to treat loss of appetite, liver and gallbladder complaints, and dyspepsia. In Europe the entire plant is used as an antispasmodic, emmenagogue, tonic, carminative, and digestive aid and for wound healing. Infusion of the aerial parts is used as a carminative, digestive aid, tonic, and emmenagogue. Wound healing is facilitated by an infusion in distilled water and application as a wash to the wound site. It is used to flavor many liqueurs.

CAUTION: Drinking the tea and applying the herb can increase sensitivity to light (photosensitivity). The tea may contain small amount of thujone, a carcinogen and liver toxin. Allergic reactions are possible, as is true of all plants. Due to its uterine-stimulating propensity, do not take yarrow internally while pregnant or nursing.

Notes: This herb should be in everyone's garden. Yarrow is one of the secret ingredients in fine beers. The bitter tea is a good digestive and anti-inflammatory that may protect you against infection when you have been exposed to infective organisms or infected individuals. I use lard for oil extractions from this herb, because lard penetrates deeper than olive and other plant-based oils.

Wildlife/veterinary uses: Leaves and stems are smudged as a mosquito repellent. Whole aerial parts are used to preserve fish by stuffing them in the fish's cleaned body cavity. Yarrow is an ingredient in Brain Cool, a herbal formulation that reportedly helps rebuild damaged nerves in horses. Some training mixes for horses contain the herb, and the supplement called Joint Support contains yarrow.

Mullein
Verbascum thapsis L.

Description: A biennial to 6 feet in height. Flower spike borne on a stout, tall stem that arises from a base whorl of woolly leaves. Leaves to 15 inches in length, ovate, covered with gray hair; basal leaves larger; clasping upper leaves less dense, smaller. Flowers yellow, ¾ to 1 inch, densely packed on a spike at apex of the stem.

Location: Nationwide. Waste ground, roadsides, fields, railroad right-of-ways.

Food: I have eaten the flowers sparingly in salads.

Traditional uses: Tea treated upper respiratory tract conditions, coughs, congestion, and infections. Used for treating bronchitis and tracheitis. Flower is an Appalachian folk remedy for treating necrotic ulcer of a recluse spider bite: Folk practitioners pounded flowers into a blend of vinegar and Epsom salts and washed the bite ten or twelve times per

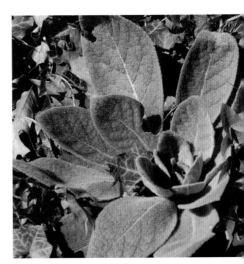

Mullein, *Verbascum thapsis*

day. Leaf and flower infusion was used to reduce and thin mucus formation. Dried leaves were smoked to stop hiccups and to induce coughing up of phlegm (expectorant). Mullein was often combined with other expectorants, such as thyme (*Thymus vulgaris*) and coltsfoot (*Tussilago farfara*). Native Americans made a necklace of the roots to be worn by teething babies. Decoction of leaves was used for colds; a raw, crushed-leaf poultice was applied over wounds and painful swellings and the mucilaginous leaves were rubbed over rashes. Mullein is said to be helpful in reducing pain from stinging nettle.

Modern uses: Commission E–approved for bronchitis and coughs. Flowers infused in olive oil are used in Europe to treat hemorrhoids and ear infections. Therapeutic teas are available over the counter.

Notes: My wife, Jill, suffers from allergies and asthma. She has used the tea of mullein leaf as an antispasmodic. Pour 1 cup of boiling water over 1 tablespoon of dried, crushed, or powdered leaves; when the mixture is room temperature, strain and drink. Add a couple plants to your yard. Simply find a first year's growth—a basal rosette of fuzzy leaves—dig it out, and transplant. The next year the biennial will bloom. The flower is striking.

Wildlife/veterinary uses: For insect and Appalachian recluse spider bite treatment, infuse whole fresh flowers in olive oil. Pack the flowers into a small jar and cover with olive oil. Let the oil and flowers infuse in the refrigerator for at least three days. Apply the warmed oil over the bite or sting every hour for twelve hours. To treat your pet's ear infection, Dummies.com suggests using a garlic-mullein ear oil, 3 to 4 drops two times daily (for details see www.dummies.com).

Burdock, Gobo Burdock
Arctium lappa L.

Description: Biennial. Mature plant many branched and spreading; to 7 or 8 feet in height, often much smaller. First year's growth sprouts broad elephant ear–like leaves (heart shaped) directly from a deep taproot. Second-year leaves are slightly smaller. Flowers crimson, with inward curving bracts that eventually form the mature seed capsule, which is a burr. This is the plant that deposits burrs on your dog and your trousers.

Location: Northern Hemisphere, temperate zone. Gardens, roadsides, just about every place you walk your dog.

Food: Harvest roots in autumn or the spring of the first year's growth. Root may be 20 or more inches long. Peel the root, then slice diagonally (julienne) and stir-fry, steam, or sauté. First year's leaves may be peeled, cooked, and eaten. Second-year flower spikes are cut and peeled and then sautéed or steamed.

Traditional uses: Historically burdock has been used to treat immune system deficiency and skin conditions. Leaf infusion was used for chronic skin problems. Root oil is used the same way; you can prepare the oil by soaking the chopped root in olive oil in the refrigerator for one

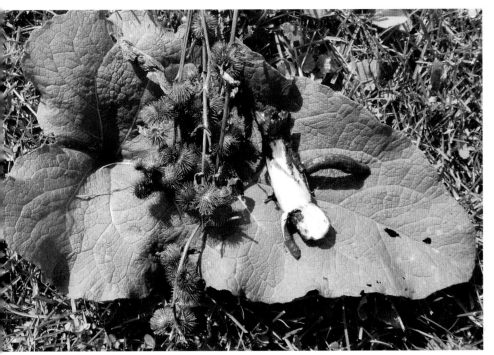

Burdock, *Arctium lappa*

month. Eating the lightly cooked root helps regulate blood sugar and is considered antidiabetic. Root polysaccharides purportedly lower blood sugar by slowing the absorption of glucose from the intestines. Drinking the root tea and eating the root are said to help treat acne. The root as food is a warming tonic and detoxifier said to strengthen the stomach, liver, and lymphatic system.

Modern uses: According to Japanese studies, the root is anticancer (antimutagenic) in animal studies. Chinese practitioners use leafy second-year branches in infusion to treat rheumatism, arthritis, and measles. This medicinal tea is often sweetened with raw cane sugar. Much of the hoopla over this herb has not been proven. Clinical trials with humans are lacking in the literature. Tincture of seeds

has been used for treating psoriasis, but personally it did not help me. The essential oil from the seed was reported to encourage hair growth and improve skin condition (not proven).

CAUTION: Avoid if pregnant or lactating.

Notes: To make a carbohydrate-rich broth, wash the first year's roots, then pound or macerate them in warm water to release the polysaccharides, inulin, and mucilage. I have eaten copious amounts of the stir-fried root, but raw root polysaccharides are difficult to digest. The root is called *gobo* in Oriental markets and runs as high as $6 a pound. It's free from your backyard if you plant it there. Simply pull burrs off a dog or your trousers, crush the burrs to release the seeds, and spread the seeds on scuffed soil in November. Plant thickly. Thin and spread seedlings in May. By the way, burdock's seed-dispersal mechanism is said to have led to the invention of Velcro.

Wildlife/veterinary uses: Brain Cool contains burdock, and the supplement manufacturer claims the product rebuilds damaged nerves in horses.

Chicory
Cichorium intybus L.

Description: Biennial or perennial to 4 feet in height. Stem erect, with few branches. Lance-shaped leaves in a basal whorl as well as additional smaller upper leaves. Blue flowers (rarely white or pink) with square tipped rays. Dandelion-like root.

Location: Nationwide. Roadsides, fields, meadow, waste ground.

Food: Chicory root is dried, roasted, mixed with coffee beans, and then ground to yield Cajun coffee. The flower petals are slightly bitter and add a nice flavor contrast when stirred into cottage cheese (let the blossoms infuse into the cheese overnight in the refrigerator). The slightly bitter flowers are healthful additions to salads, jump-starting the digestion process.

Traditional uses: The root dried or fresh is decocted in water as a diuretic, dietetic, and laxative. Root tea stimulates digestion, improving both peristalsis and absorption. Root decoction was used externally to treat fever blisters. Cherokees used root infusion as a tonic for the nerves (nervine).

Modern uses: Commission E–approved for stimulating appetite and treating or

alleviating dyspepsia. Homeopathic practitioners use it for gallbladder and liver complaints. Root decoction may reduce blood sugar. Root constituents are antibacterial in vitro. Chicory's anti-inflammatory activity is being studied. Root extract may slow heart rate and reduce heart contractility. Animal studies showed a cholesterol-lowering effect. In India the root decoction is used to treat headaches, vomiting, and diarrhea.

Notes: This is a must-have, attractive garden flower with edible leaves, edible flowers, and a stimulating root. The leaf extraction is not as bitter and evokes a milder response than the root decoction.

Wildlife/veterinary uses: Chicory is particularly beneficial when fed to lambs in late spring and summer to spur high animal growth rates so that lambs meet prime lamb specifications for domestic and export markets. Trials have shown that prime lambs consistently have high live weight gains when grazing on chicory and white clover forage compared to

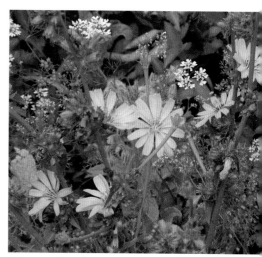

Chicory, *Cichorium intybus*

either perennial ryegrass/subclover or tall fescue/subclover pastures. Animal studies showed that eating chicory slows heart rate.

Dock, Yellow Dock, Curly Dock
Rumex crispus L.

Description: Perennial with large, wavy basal leaves broadly (and sometimes narrowly) lance shaped with a sour to bitter taste. Flower spikes to 3 feet, with green flowers located on heads, several clusters per long bloom stalk. Blooms May to September. Root large, deep, yellowish.

Location: Nationwide. Fringes of yards, streamsides, vacant lots, roadsides.

Food: Young leaves may be steamed, sautéed, or stir-fried. Be judicious, as leaves may be bitter. Try steaming the herbs, then frying them in olive oil. The inner pulp of the flowering stem is eaten after cooking. Squeeze pulp from the skin to reduce bitterness. Seeds are plentiful and may be gathered and made into a mush.

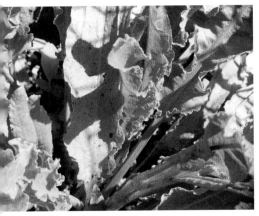

Curly dock, *Rumex crispus*

Traditional uses: Native Americans mashed the root and applied it to the skin to treat arthritis. Cherokees used the root juice to treat diarrhea. One unusual use was rubbing the throat with a crushed leaf to treat sore throat. Cooked seeds were eaten to stem diarrhea. Dried and powdered root was used to stop bleeding (styptic). Pioneers considered the plant to be an excellent blood purifier, a spring tonic for whatever ails you.

Modern uses: Naturopaths simmer the sliced root and administer the broth to pregnant women as a source of iron without the constipation that results from taking elemental iron supplements. The bitter taste of the herb (root and leaves) stimulates digestion: It increases hydrochloric acid secretion, increases peristalsis, and improves secretion of other digestive enzymes. The whole plant in decoction is said to cleanse toxins from body and may have a laxative effect because of inherent tannins and anthraquinones (fights constipation). Reported to help improve chronic skin problems. Bitter taste stimulates liver activity (blood purifier) and may help cleanse the liver, thereby relieving related skin manifestations. Dock is sometimes combined with dandelion root to treat skin problems.

CAUTION: Restrict the amount of dock leaves you eat because of the high tannin and oxalic acid content. These chemicals may be harmful to the kidneys when eaten in excess.

Notes: Yellow dock or curly dock plants savage my garden. I dig them up and throw the lot on my mulch pile, where they take hold and grow some more. The plant scrubs minerals from the soil, providing a soil-enriching mulch. Simmer the root (fresh or dried) and steal the minerals for yourself. Spaniards eat the plant for its vitamin C content and use it as a mild laxative and diuretic.

Wildlife/veterinary uses: Yellow dock tea is taken to treat insect bites, stings, and insect-vectored diseases. Yellow dock is an integral part of an antiflea formula (see flea article at www.allourpets.com for more details).

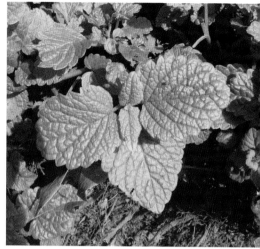

Lemon balm, *Melissa officinalis*

Lemon Balm, Balm Melissa

Melissa officinalis L.

Description: Many-branched perennial to 2 or 3 feet in height, aromatic. Stems erect, square, hairy to hairless. Leaves have petioles and are oval to rhomboid shaped and plentiful. Leaves lemon scented to the touch. Produces small, white, two-lipped flowers on the end of an upcurved corolla tube. Flowers localized in one-sided false whorls in upper axils of leaves. Seeds are nut brown. Blooms in summer.

Location: A garden plant that escapes from garden to roadsides, waste ground. Ask your herb-growing friends to show you this plant. Available at garden stores. Worth having.

Food: Use flowers and leaf buds in salads, desserts, and toppings and cooked with vegetables. Mature, aromatic balm leaves can be used in baths. Infuse as a tea or as an ice cream (remove leaves before freezing). A cold infusion with other mints is excellent: Stuff a jar with lemon balm leaves, other mint leaves of all kinds, thyme leaves, and two slices of lemon. Put in the refrigerator overnight. Adding the thyme leaves make this a must-have tea for mountaineers, as it protects them from mountain sickness.

Traditional uses: Phytochemicals in lemon balm may relax muscles in the autonomic system of the digestive tract and uterus. More research is needed to confirm this. In Chinese traditional medicine lemon balm cooling is in the second degree, like chamomile, mint, valerian, passionflower; it is a relaxing nervine, a central nervous system relaxant, and a calming agent. The first leaves of spring and flowers of summer may be dried. In China 1 to 4 grams of dried aerial parts are taken in decoction three times per day to treat stress. Lemon balm is a peripheral vasodilator and is cooling to fevers and was historically used to reduce blood pressure (unproven). It's traditionally considered a longevity drug.

Modern uses: Commission E–approved for insomnia and nervous agitation. German studies suggest that citral and citronellal in lemon balm relax the central nervous system. Polyphenolic compounds are antiviral, used specifically on herpes simplex (cold sores).

CAUTION: Lemon balm may inhibit thyroid function. Naturopaths use it to treat overactive thyroid. Not to be used in pregnant or lactating women, as it is considered a uterine stimulant.

Notes: Lemon balm can be an aggressive garden herb, at first rewarding and then a nuisance. I cannot drink enough tea to keep up with it. But I can't live without it either—like my wife, my daughter, and my golden retriever.

Wildlife/veterinary uses: The chemical eugenol in lemon balm is a chemoattractant to Japanese beetles. The concentrated oil can be purchased in the first-aid section of some drugstores. Put the eugenol on a piece of absorbent cloth and fashion a trap from a bottle (see the Japanese beetle traps at your local garden center for construction ideas). Flowers from this mint family plant are sought by bees, butterflies, and hummingbirds.

Milkweed, Common Milkweed
Asclepias syriaca L.

Description: Perennial to 4 feet in height. Single stem. Leaves opposite, large, elliptical, to 8 inches in length. Pink flowers in drooping clusters grow from leaf axils. Seedpod is striking, Arabian slipperlike.

Location: Various species found nationwide. Edges of cornfields, waste ground, roadsides, railroad right-of-ways, meadows, dune lands, gardens.

Food: Native Americans prepared *A. syriaca* shoots like asparagus. Pick the shoots before the milky sap appears, simmer in two changes of water, then sauté in oil. Flower buds are prepared like cooked broccoli when harvested before they open. Flowers buds and seedpods are prepared as follows: Boil water, pour over seedpods, let water and pods steep for five minutes, then pour off the water. Repeat by pouring a second boil of water over the once-steeped pods, pour off the water, then stir-fry in olive oil or butter. Many people use *three* water baths over the pods, and that is recommended for your first encounter with the plant. The flowers may be dried and stored for winter use in soups and stews. Flowers have

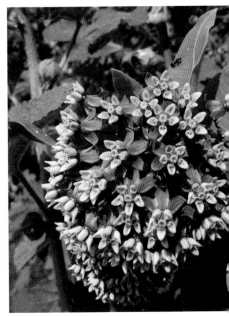
Milkweed, *Asclepias syriaca*

been diced, sweetened, and made into marmalade. Native Americans ground seeds into flour.

Traditional uses: Native Americans pounded or split the roots for drying. Dried roots in decoction have a mild cardiac-stimulating effect—without the toxic effects of digitalis. Be warned this should be practiced with medical supervision because *A. syriaca* contains toxic cardiac glycosides and requires careful preparation before use. Native Americans believed the plant promoted milk flow (lactagogue) because of the milky white sap, a belief in keeping with the Doctrine of Signatures, which states that "like treats like." Latex from the leaves was rubbed on warts and, reportedly, on cancerous tumors. Native American lore suggests that approximately a fistful (1½ cups) of milkweed was dried and pounded to a pulp, then mixed with three dried *Arisaema* (jack-in-the-pulpit) rhizomes. The plants were then put in a skin or gourd and infused into water for twenty or thirty minutes. The milkweed and jack-in-the-pulpit infusion was swallowed 1 cup per hour to induce sterility. All varieties of milkweed were used as a poultice by First Peoples to treat wounds. The white gum was applied over insect stings, bites, and spider envenomations. Root infusion was used for kidney ailments, and the dried leaves were infused for stomach problems. Native Americans also used the white sap of the plant to treat poison ivy, ringworm, and other skin problems. The boiled root decoction was used externally for edema and ringworm and internally for congestive heart failure and kidney disorders. The eclectics used

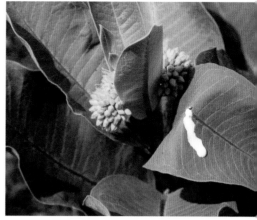

Milkweed leaves and sap

dried and powdered milkweed root in a tea for asthma and as a mild sedative.

Modern uses: Homeopathic preparations of milkweed treat many ailments, including edema, dropsy, and dysmenorrhea (as an emmenagogue). *A. curassavica* from China is used to disperse fever (clears heat), improve blood circulation, and control bleeding. The entire plant is dried and decocted as a cardiac tonic. Other Chinese formulations are used for tonsillitis, pneumonia, bronchitis, urethritis, and externally for wounds. According to herbalist Michael Moore, the dried gum may be chewed in small portions as an expectorant to treat a dry cough; the bitterness stimulates saliva flow.

CAUTION: Keep in mind I have only eaten *A. syriaca*. Other species may be toxic. Do not experiment with milkweed species without expert guidance from a licensed holistic health-care practitioner. *A. syriaca* contains toxic cardiac glycosides and requires careful preparation before use (see the food section, above). Root decoction may be emetic, and it may stimulate the heart. A few people may get allergic reactions from the milky sap. According to Steven Foster and James Duke in *A Field Guide to Medicinal Plants: Eastern and Central North America* (see appendix D), the plant is considered "dangerous and contraceptive."

Notes: You can gather milkweed resin by cutting leaves and stems, working your way down from the top of the plant. For example, cut a leaf stem or stem near the top of plant, then scrape away the white resin. When the plant wound dries and skins over, cut a bit farther down on the plant and collect more resin. The collected resin will oxidize and dry in a glass or stainless collecting dish. Stir or turn it occasionally for thorough drying. This process does not kill the plant as long as you leave ample leaves and stem for it to survive. Milkweed seed fiber and seed hair was once used as life-jacket batting. The fragrant flowers are sweet, a potential source of sugar. I transplanted three varieties of domestic milkweed to my garden so I could watch them parade their striking beauty year-round. My daughter uses the milky latex of the leaves and stems to glue paper. The strong, fibrous stems can be made into cordage, and the pulp may be chopped, shredded, boiled, and prepared into paper.

Wildlife/veterinary uses: Milkweed plants are exotic looking in a garden context. They attract bees, butterflies (monarchs, fritillaries), and hummingbirds. With luck you will soon see monarch caterpillars crawling over the leaves. Watch out for black and yellow sucking insects called milkweed bugs (*Oncopeltus*

fasciatus) on the underside of leaves. Be careful when eating milkweed pods that the bug is not in there waiting for you.

Red Clover
Trifolium pratense L.

Description: Perennial to 12 to 18 inches in height. Three leaves with distinct V marking on each leaflet. Leaflets fine toothed, ovate. Flowers pink to red, dome shaped or rounded.

Location: Nationwide. Fields, roadsides, waste ground in full sun.

Food: Red clover makes a relaxing floral tea. Florets may be tossed on salads. The tea is made from the fresh or dried flower.

Traditional uses: Floral tea was traditionally used as a cure-all. Decoction or tea used as an external wash on burns, wounds, and insect bites. Pioneers claimed that drinking the tea purified the blood, an enervating tonic. Tea is considered an expectorant as therapy for respiratory problems such as asthma,

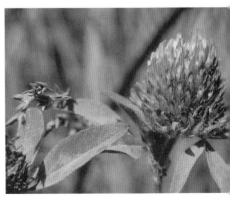

Red clover, *Trifolium pratense*

bronchitis, and whooping cough and as an antispasmodic and mild sedative. Dried flower heads are traditionally considered anticancer and are part of the Hoxley and Essiac anticancer formula, which includes red clover, sheep sorrel, burdock root, slippery elm bark, rhubarb root, watercress, blessed thistle, and kelp. Red clover is also used as a wash for psoriasis and eczema. Isoflavone estrogen-like compounds in clover are used to treat menopausal and postmenopausal problems.

Modern uses: A red clover isoflavone concentrate in tablet form reduced bone loss in a double-blind placebo controlled trial with 177 women between the ages of forty-nine and sixty-five (see Atkinson, Compston, Day, et al. in appendix D). A smaller trial showed that red clover derivatives reduced hot flashes (see Van de Weijeer, Barentsen; appendix D). And a third study showed a 23 percent increase in arterial blood flow to the heart in women (see Nestel, Pomeroy, Kay, et al.; appendix D). Red clover is still used to treat menopausal symptoms and may improve blood flow in the heart.

CAUTION: Standardized red clover extracts should be used and even then only under the supervision of a licensed health-care practitioner. The drug may increase bleeding and has other side effects.

Notes: Floral teas should be used sparingly or not at all, unless supervised by a holistic health-care professional.

Wildlife/veterinary uses: Red clover is an important forage for game and domestic animals. It is a nitrogen-fixing soil replenisher. A trial with female sheep grazing on clover showed that viscosity of the cervix is affected and may reduce fertility.

Lamb's-quarters, Goosefoot; Epazote
Chenopodium album L.;
C. ambrosioides L.

Description: Lamb's-quarters (*C. album*) is an annual to 5 feet in height. Light green or grayish green young leaves with powderlike substance beneath, three lobed, with a goosefoot or diamond shape. Small green flowers in clusters grow from top third of plant and many of the branches. Seeds gray colored. *C. ambrosioides* grows to 5 feet. Green to yellow green, toothed leaves. Green flowers and seeds borne on aromatic terminal spikes with a light fragrance of sweet turpentine.

Location: Nationwide. Meadows, roadsides, gardens, waste ground, edges of cultivated fields. Epazote is more southern in its range—Texas, Mexico, Arizona—but will self-seed in temperate gardens.

Food: I add lamb's-quarters leaves to salads and stir-fries and use it inside steamed wontons rolled in quinoa seeds, carrots, and burdock root. Seeds may be ground and used in baking recipes. Epazote leaves are strong; use them sparingly to flavor corn, bean, and fish dishes; soups; and cooked vegetable dishes.

Traditional uses: Lamb's-quarter tea was used to treat stomachache, scurvy, and diarrhea, and the leaves were used as a poultice over wounds and bites. In

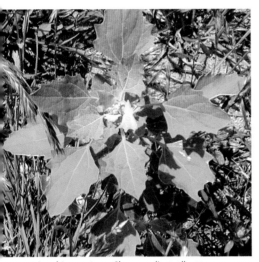
Lamb's-quarters, *Chenopodium album*

Mexico the cooked leaves and seed heads are believed to keep the digestive system clean and healthy. Cree Indians used the leaves for arthritis and rheumatism by washing the joints and limbs with the decoction. Inuit people believe the leaves when cooked with beans dispel gas. The Iroquois used a cold infusion of the plant to treat diarrhea. Leaves are high in vitamin C content (used to treat scurvy) and, when eaten with their seeds, form a complete essential amino acid. The tea of epazote, like that of lamb's-quarters, is considered a spring tonic and fever reducer. A warm poultice of the leaves is used to treat headache.

Modern uses: Traditional uses are still employed. Epazote is found in virtually every Mexican kitchen as a spice and medicinal.

CAUTION: The phytochemicals in epazote are potentially toxic in overdose. Use epazote as a spice in small amounts: Three or four leaves to 2 quarts of beans,

or a couple of crushed leaves to a bowl of soup. But no more.

Notes: I grow lamb's-quarters in my garden. *C. quinoa,* an edible primal grain, can be purchased in health-food stores and at Seventh-day Adventist markets. Eat a few seeds and plant the rest. My book *Basic Essentials Edible Wild Plants* offers lamb's-quarters recipes and information on related edible species.

Wildlife/veterinary uses: Both lamb's-quarters and epazote are considered antihelminthic (antiworm) and are used as worming agents (vermifuge) with animals. Put the aerial parts of the whole herb in your pet's doghouse or in its bedding. The two species are used as fumigants against mosquitoes and as soil-based larvae inhibitors for lawns.

Catnip
Nepeta cataria L.

Description: Perennial to 3½ feet in height. Erect and many-branched stems. Leaves grayish, giving plant a whitish gray appearance. Leaves 1 to 3 inches, ovate, serrated, with gray underside. Leaf petiole to 1½ inches long. Flower spike has large cluster of individual flowers attached with short pedicles.

Location: Nationwide. Gardens, roadsides, and waste ground. Tolerates well-drained, dry areas.

Food: Leaves and flowers are used fresh or dried, in tea as a relaxing drink or treatment.

Traditional uses: Aerial parts of the plant in infusion are a bitter, astringent, and cooling antispasmodic. Catnip leaf and flower teas provide a mild sedative effect. It is antiflatulent and may settle a colicky baby; check with your holistic health-care professional before using it in this manner. It can be used to soothe the digestive tract, and it may provide relief from menstrual cramps by mildly stimulating menstruation. The herbal tea promotes sweating, thereby lowering fever in acute infections. Like many herbal teas, it is a mild diuretic.

Modern uses: Naturopaths use catnip to treat colic and stomachache in children. According to Andrew Chevallier in the *Encyclopedia of Medicinal Plants,* catnip may be tinctured and used as a rub for rheumatic and arthritic joints. The tea is also used to stimulate the gallbladder. Naturopaths combine catnip leaves with elderberry flowers for treating acute infections. Another combination as a sleep aid is catnip, valerian root, and hops. This combination is used to reduce stress and as a relaxant.

CAUTION: Not to be used during pregnancy.

Notes: Catnip is one of my favorite teas. I prefer it prepared from the fresh herb in a cold infusion, as its physiologically active constituents are volatile and reduced by drying. Typical dosage is 3 cups per day. This plant is a cat's drug of choice, so start catnip indoors and transplant it when it is at least a foot tall. Maybe then it will survive the onslaught of drug-seeking felines! Actinidine, an iridoid glycoside, is the cat-stimulating part of the plant.

Wildlife/veterinary uses: Catnip is a feline stimulant and intoxicant but a human calming agent. Catnip is formulated into training mixes for horses. A canine catnip stimulant in a pump spray is available by catalog—Google it.

Echinacea, Purple Coneflower
Echinacea purpurea (L.) Moench; *E. angustifolia* DC.

Description: Erect perennial to 2½ feet in height. Leaves large, opposite or alternate, with smooth margins and rough surface. Rhizome (root) when sliced shows yellowish center flecked with black, covered in thin barklike skin. Purple blossoms large, solitary, with spreading rays. Bracts rigid, with thornlike tips.

Location: Eastern and central United States. Meadows and prairies, fringes of fields and parks. Will grow in gardens nationwide.

Traditional uses: Root and flowers were used as a snakebite treatment. Boiled

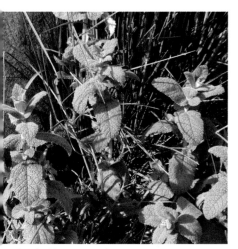
Catnip, *Nepeta cataria*

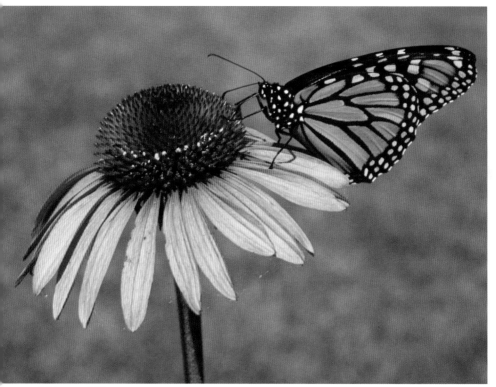

Echinacea, *Echinacea purpurea*

root water was used to treat sore throats. Mashed plant was applied to wounds as a therapy for infections. Root infusion was once considered a treatment for gonorrhea. Masticated root was held on sore tooth to treat infection.

Modern uses: Commercial preparations of roots, leaves, and flowers are used to treat colds, flu, coughs, bronchitis, fever, urinary infections, inflammations of the mouth and pharynx, weakened immune function, and wounds and burns. Echinacea therapy is considered useful if started immediately at the onset of upper respiratory infections, taken three times a day and continued until the person is well. Echinacea enhances immunity in several ways. Polysaccharide-initiated response follows a bell curve: steep initial activity, improving immune response up to 32 percent. Then response peaks and after four to six days tapers off. Therefore echinacea is used for acute instead of chronic conditions. Note that a recent study challenged echinacea's immune-modulating effect (Schwartz et al., "Oral Administration of Freshly Pressed Juice of Echinacea . . . ," *Phytomedicine* 12 [2005]: 625–31).

Echinacea is also taken internally to treat skin diseases, fungal infections (both *Candida* and *Listeria*), and slow-healing wounds, boils, gangrene, upper respiratory tract infections, and sinusitis.

Used externally for acne and psoriasis (not proven by this sufferer). Root oil has inhibited leukemia cells in vitro and vivo studies.

CAUTION: A study of 412 pregnant Canadian women (206 of whom took echinacea during pregnancy) showed that spontaneous abortions were twice as frequent in the echinacea group, including thirteen spontaneous abortions. Consult your physician before using echinacea while pregnant. The herb should be avoided by those allergic to plants in the aster/daisy family and by those with active autoimmune disease.

Notes: I have prepared and used an alcohol tincture of *E. purpurea* flowers as a gargle for mouth and tongue ulcers. I use it to prevent colds and the flu. Commercial extracts come in solid and liquid standardized form with recommended dosage. A few years ago I had a staphylococcus infection (cellulitis), an imbedded cyst in my buttock. My physician suggested that I have it cut out before it burst open and infected other parts of my body. I begged to try the echinacea floral extraction. The large cystlike infection disappeared in three days and has not returned. I continued the therapy for a total of six days.

Wildlife/veterinary uses: Echinacea is used in all my pigeon-racing formulas as a health-protecting and cleansing agent after races. Bees and butterflies flit and flip over this flower. It is an ingredient in a natural product to rebuild damaged nerves in horses. Many herbalists who treat animals use echinacea to treat acute infections in pets (see www.petsage.com).

Bee Balm; Wild Bergamot, Horsemint

Monarda didyma L.; *M. fistulosa* L.

Description: Perennial of the mint family, to 3 feet in height. Straight stem grooved, hard. Oval to lance-shaped leaves in pairs, rough on both sides. Both species have flowers in one to three false whorls; flowers are horn shaped—pluck one and notice their resemblance to a stork's head and neck. *M. didyma* has red flowers; *M. fistulosa* has blue flowers. Red *M. didyma* florets taste pineapple-like, weakly oregano flavored, whereas *M. fistulosa* has a strong oregano flavor.

Location: *M. didyma* is readily found in wet areas from Georgia through Michigan into Canada. *M. fistulosa* is found across the nation, often along trails in the Rockies and Cascades and roadsides in Michigan, Indiana, and throughout the East, usually in well-drained areas, but it will tolerate wet and dryness.

Food: Eat young leaves raw, cook leaves with other dishes for flavoring, add flowers to salads or in tea. Either species is

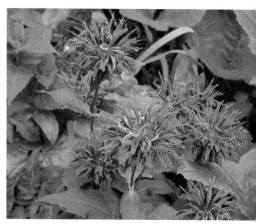

Bee balm, *Monarda didyma*

excellent as a garnish over sauces, especially Italian (*fistulosa* is oregano flavored, strong, whereas *didyma* is milder, pineapple flavored). Use both species to season meats for drying and/or smoking. Add *M. fistulosa* flowers to black tea to get an Earl Grey–like flavor.

Traditional uses: *M. didyma* is steeped in hot water to make Oswego tea. *M. fistulosa* is stronger tasting, with a flavor like oregano. Both plants were used by Native Americans as a carminative, abortifacient, cold remedy, sedative, analgesic, hemostat, emetic, pulmonary aid, and diaphoretic and to treat coughs, induce sweating, and treat the flu. Navajos considered *M. fistulosa* to be lightning medicine and gunshot medicine—powerful warrior plants. Pioneers used it to treat bronchial complaints, sinusitis, digestive problems, and flatulence and as an anti-rheumatic and expectorant. At one time *M. didyma* was used as a alternative to quinine.

Modern uses: *M. didyma* is most widely used. Its chemical constituents may provide protection from diseases of aging. Aerial parts in infusion have chemicals that may prevent acetylcholine (neural transmitter) breakdown. Modern holistic practitioners use the plant to treat menstrual cramps and other symptoms of premenstrual syndrome and as a digestive and antiflatulent.

CAUTION: Not to be used during pregnancy. If you have flower allergies, be careful when using bee balm flowers in salads and teas—although there have been no documented side effects.

Notes: I eat up to twenty florets per day. Teas should contain ten to twenty flowers for full flavor. I prefer *M. didyma* over *M. fistulosa* for salads and as a garnish. *M. fistulosa* is best in sauces where an oregano flavor is preferred.

Wildlife/veterinary uses: Both of these perennials should be in your garden to attract beneficial insects. The red-flowered *M. didyma* will attract hummingbirds. A poultice or infusion of bee balm, plantain, sage, mullein, calendula, or chamomile can be directly applied to a pet directly at the site of an insect bite or sting. A skin rinse of bee balm, chamomile, peppermint, catnip, or thyme may bring relief from pain in a dog or cat. For more on these herbal tips for pets, go to www.bowtiepress.com/bowtie/xrptherb.asp.

Evening Primrose
Oenothera biennis L.

Description: Biennial to 3 feet or taller. Fleshy, turniplike root. First-year plant: nonflowering basal rosette of leaves. Second year: erect, blooming plant, conspicuous in the fall with large seed-filled fruit capsules. Oblong, lance-shaped leaves, pointed and finely dentate. Fragrant, bugle-shaped yellow flowers, 1 inch long, growing from leaf axils. Flowers open in evening. Fruit linear-oblong, four sided, downy, about ½ to 1 inch in length, containing dark gray to black seeds with sharp edges.

Location: Several species found nationwide. Desert fringe to alpine meadows;

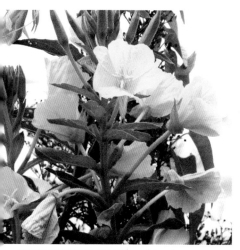

Evening primrose, *Oenothera biennis*

gardens, roadsides, waste ground, fields, prairies.

Food: The root is edible (the first-year root is best). New leaves of first or second year are edible in salads or stir-fries. The leaves are tough and need to be cooked. Seeds can be poured out of seed capsule. The seed capsule looks like a small, dried okra pod. Immature seed capsules may be cooked like okra, but they taste nothing like okra.

Traditional uses: Native Americans used warm root poultices to treat piles. Roots were chewed to increase strength and endurance. The whole plant was bruised, soaked, and used as a poultice on bruises and sores.

Modern uses: The seed oil is used to treat essential fatty acid deficiency and to lower cholesterol. A cholesterol-lowering effect was not shown in a 1986 study but did prove effective in a double-blind crossover study conducted in 1996. Seed extract is said to dilate coronary arteries

and clear arterial obstruction. Used as a holistic treatment for intermittent claudication. Other uses include treatments of atopic eczema and psoriasis (not effective with this author). Oil may provide relief from PMS symptoms, although one study disputed this claim. One study showed that in women who had recurrent breast cysts, evening primrose oil (EPO) treatment resulted in a slightly lower rate of recurrence as compared to placebo. The essential fatty acids and amino acids in the seeds are reportedly good for treating mild depression. EPO has been used successfully with vitamin B6 therapy to treat breast pain (mastalgia). The oil is considered anticoagulant, demulcent, and a precursor of prostaglandin E (anti-inflammatory).

Another study suggests that EPO may reverse neurological damage in diabetic patients. It provided significantly increased serum essential fatty acids in insulin-dependent children. EPO therapy may improve liver function in alcoholics and is said to decrease the use of nonsteroidal anti-inflammatory drugs in treatment for rheumatoid arthritis.

CAUTION: In large doses EPO may cause headache, diarrhea, indigestion, and nausea. Researchers recommend not using evening primrose oil in cases of schizophrenia and/or with epileptogenic drugs (phenothiazines). No long-term studies have been performed to determine its effects during pregnancy and lactation.

Notes: Evening primrose oil is high in GLA, a naturally occurring nutrient that is also found in breast milk. This widely used nutritional supplement has been marketed for more than thirty years. My wife takes evening primrose oil for treating PMS. She feels it helps; my observation is that it helps minimally. I have psoriasis and have found this oil and borage oil to be expensive and ineffective treatments. I have more success at less cost using fish-oil capsules.

Wildlife/veterinary uses: Seeds are fine additions to bird feeders. Finches, sparrows, and numerous other birds will be attracted to the seed-laden capsules of the plants. Omega-6 essential fatty acids from evening primrose are a constituent in Healthy Coat Skin & Coat Tabs from the Doctors Foster and Smith catalog (www.drsfostersmith.com).

Butterfly Milkweed, Pleurisy Root
Asclepias tuberosa L.

Description: Perennial to 30 inches in height. Tuberous root, grooved along its length, with root hairs. Leaves alternate, hairless, oblong, and deep green. Flowers orange, numerous, on panicles at the top of the flower stem. This milkweed does not have the latex found in other species.

Location: Much of North America: in the East north of the Mason-Dixon Line, in the Four Corners area of the West, and north into Canada. Commonly used as a garden ornamental.

Food: Not edible.

Traditional uses: This is a premier Native American expectorant medicine. The root was used in decoction for treating pleurisy, bronchitis, gastritis, influenza, pneumonia, colds, and asthma. It was used to reduce fever by causing perspiration. It was also used to treat uterine disorders (dysmenorrhea), and therefore its use is contraindicated for pregnant women. The mashed root was applied externally as a poultice, whereas the mashed root in infusion was indicated for treating snakebites, bruises, rheumatism, wounds, and weeping ulcers. The dried-leaf poultice was wrapped around snakebites.

Modern uses: Medicinal properties of the plant are untested and unproven. It is still used by Native Americans and herbalists but has not been tested in double-blind, placebo-controlled, randomized studies.

CAUTION: Never to be used during pregnancy. A high dose of the extraction is emetic. Use only under the supervision of

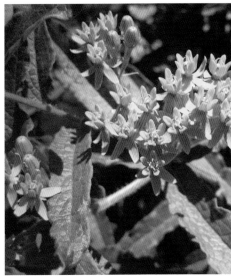

Butterfly milkweed, *Asclepias tuberosa*

a trained and licensed holistic health-care practitioner.

Notes: Locate this colorful herb up front—along garden edges and walkways—where it can show off in your garden. It is short and spreading and can get lost behind larger plants.

Wildlife/veterinary uses: An attractive and fragrant bee, butterfly, and hummingbird magnet. The monarch butterfly requires milkweed for its egg laying and larvae nutrition. Whorled milkweed (*A. subverticillata*), which has severely whorled leaves, has been indicated to cause sudden death by toxin in cattle.

Motherwort
Leonurus cardiaca L.

Description: Perennial in the mint family. Erect, to 3½ feet in height, often shorter. Stem quadrangular, grooved, usually hairy and hollow. Opposite leaves on long petiole; leaves deeply lobed, coarsely toothed; upper leaves with three to five lobes, dark green on top, light green underneath. Small red flowers present in dense false whorls in the upper leaf axils. Flowers from April to August, depending on latitude and altitude. Plant leaves when crushed have an unusual smell.

Location: Introduced and has spread nationwide. Waste ground, roadsides, edges of lawns.

Food: Although it is not considered a food, a few holistic practitioners will consume the seeds for their beta-carotene and essential fatty acids content.

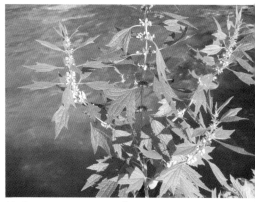

Motherwort, *Leonurus cardiaca*

Traditional uses: Traditionally used by the Chinese and by pioneers to tone heart muscle. (*Leonurus cardiaca* means "lion's heart.") It was also indicated as a tonic for treating amenorrhea, dysmenorrhea, urinary cramps, and general weakness. It reportedly cleared toxins from the body. Ancient Greeks used the herb with pregnant women to treat stress and anxiety, but modern herbals warn women against using the herb during pregnancy because of its uterine-stimulating effects. Motherwort was used traditionally for stemming bacterial and fungal infections, both internally and externally. Whole aerial parts (leaves, flowers, stems) were gathered when the plant was in bloom and the infusion used to treat asthma and heart palpitations.

Modern uses: Commission E–approved for nervous-heart complaints (palpitations) and thyroid dysfunction. Homeopathic preparations treat menopause. The plant, considered by many herbalists and naturopaths as a superior woman's herb, is a uterine and circulatory stimulant that may relieve PMS. It is hypotensive, anti-spasmodic, and diuretic; it works as a laxative, a sedative, and an emmenagogue. Leonurine in the plant tones the uterine membrane (membrane regulation). A physician friend of mine has used motherwort and passionflower to lower blood pressure with his patients.

Chinese practitioners use the herb as a single herb and do not typically compound it with other herbs. *L. japonicus* is widely used in China, where its effectiveness is documented in numerous clinical studies. A decoction of dried herb is used in China as a uterine stimulant. The aqueous decoction is reported as antibacterial. Chinese treat nephritis with aqueous extract made from 180 to 240 grams of fresh herb in 1 liter of water in decoction.

CAUTION: Consuming the seeds may be uterine stimulating and should be avoided by pregnant and lactating women.

Notes: The plant grows everywhere along the edges of my yard. Folklore predicts that if you have a woman in the home, a wife or daughter, the plant appears and provides itself as medicine. It transplants readily as long as you get the entire woody root.

Wildlife/veterinary uses: Bumblebees utilize the flowers for pollen and nectar. Motherwort provides protection and habitat in prairies for field sparrows. Originally from southern Germany, the plant is considered an alien weed and is often eradicated, but not by me.

Foxglove, Purple Foxglove
Digitalis purpurea L.

Description: Biennial to 3 to 5 feet in height. Lance-shaped leaves, fuzzy (hairy) in basal rosette. When without flower stalk, the basal rosette of leaves looks somewhat like mullein leaves or comfrey leaves, rarely dock leaves, but beware—the leaves of *Digitalis* are toxic. Flowers thimble shaped, white to purple, aggregated on a spike. They look like gloves, hence the common name. Flowers bloom in the summer of the second year.

Location: Northwestern and eastern mountain states. A common mountain roadside wildflower and a favorite ornamental in gardens from coast to coast.

Food: Not edible; toxic.

Traditional uses: The powdered leaf contains potent cardiac glycosides perhaps first used by Celtic people in Europe. Overdose causes nausea, vomiting, slowed pulse, fainting, and possibly death. Used externally on wounds and

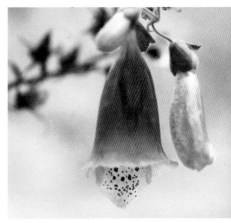

Foxglove, *Digitalis purpurea*

ulcers. Used in the British Isles to treat tumors, ulcers, headaches, and abscesses.

Modern uses: The plant-derived drug is considered obsolete. Better synthetic, pure substances are available and used. The plant contains cardiac glycosides, used to model the now-synthesized drugs that increase heartbeat strength and lower venous pressure. It lowers oxygen requirements of the heart and reduces the frequency of abnormal heartbeats (atrialfibrillation).

CAUTION: Leaves are toxic.

Notes: Transplants well to the garden and makes a striking plant. It tolerates some shade but prefers sun and well-drained soil.

Wildlife/veterinary uses: Toxic when ingested by wildlife. Foxglove is potentially fatal to cats that eat the plant. Not only is the entire foxglove plant toxic, so is the water from the vase if the flower spikes are cut and brought indoors.

Pokeweed, Poke Salad
Phytolacca americana L.

Description: Perennial to 10 feet in height, but more typically 5 feet. Thick, smooth, reddish stems when mature, stems hollow and usually marked with grooves. Root long and thick. Leaves ovate to lance shaped, alternate, 5 to 10 inches in length, with entire margins. Leaves produce a musty scent when rubbed. Flowers have five greenish white sepals, on racemes, with a calyx but no corolla. Berries borne from drooping cluster, shiny purplish to black when ripe.

Location: Missouri River east to the Atlantic coast and south to the Gulf. Waste ground, fields, roadsides, gardens.

Food: The young shoots of this plant are excellent-tasting greens, edible only in the spring. The leaves contain three times as much vitamin C as a lemon and are mineral rich. The leaves should be boiled in a change of water. Avoid pokeweed once the stem and leaf petioles have started to turn purple, because the lectin content rises as the plant matures. Cooking destroys some of the lectins, and human digestive juices get others, but be careful—your window of opportunity is short. If you are uncertain, you can find these greens canned and commercially available. Stems when young and tender may be blanched and pickled. One of my students reported eating pokeweed rather late into the season, with the flower buds on. She confessed to their potent cathartic activity. Seeds, berries, and roots are toxic. Cherokee peoples made a drink of crushed ripe berries that were mixed with sour grapes, sweetened, then strained and blended with powdered cornmeal.

Traditional uses: Native Americans traditionally used the root poultice over rheumatoid joints. Berries were made into tea to treat rheumatic condition and dysentery. Infusion of root was used to treat eczema and ulcerated wounds and to reduce swelling. Dried and powdered roots were spread over cuts and sores. The plant was used as a laxative and emetic. A decoction mixed with other plants was taken as a blood purifier and stimulant (see Moerman, *Native*

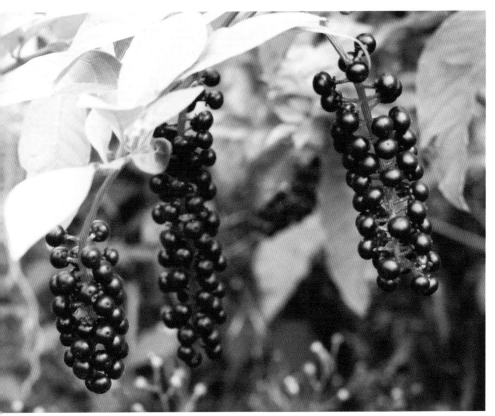

Pokeweed, *Phytolacca americana*

American Ethnobiology; appendix D). An infusion of root and branches was used in sweat lodges to produce steam that is considered antirheumatic. Root was pounded and mixed with grease and applied to bunions.

Modern uses: The plant parts are reported as purgative and antiarthritic. Antiviral proteins in leaves have been indicated as a possible treatment for cancer and viral infections. Homeopathic doses are available for rheumatism, inflammations of the mammary glands and respiratory tract, infections, and fevers. Root saponins are emetic. The root extract has demonstrated an immune-enhancing effect. Berries are used by the food industry as a coloring.

CAUTION: Overdose of pokeweed leads to diarrhea, respiratory distress, hypotension, dizziness, thirst, tachycardia, vomiting, and—if the dose is high enough—acute spasm and death. Berries are particularly toxic to children, and the ingestion of just one berry by a child is cause for concern. More than ten berries may be harmful to an adult, according to the *PDR for Herbal Medicines* (first edition).

Notes: Traditional peoples used the berries as a dye. In Appalachia the root is brought into root cellars, placed in a trough, covered with dirt, watered to induce growth, and the new edible shoots are eaten. One controversial therapy is called the pokeberry purge. It requires ingesting one berry to start a cleansing process, then taking one additional berry each day for twenty or twenty-one days (with twenty-one berries taken on the last day). I'm not interested. Too risky! Knowing me, I would end up with twenty-one days of diarrhea or worse. A fruit juice fast is a purgative more to my liking.

Wildlife/veterinary uses: Berries are eaten by birds with no ill effects.

Passionflower
Passiflora incarnata L.

Description: Numerous varieties, all somewhat similar. Perennial vine. Woody stem climbing to 30 feet or more; longitudinal striated bark when mature. Leaves alternate, with petioles, serrated with fine hair on both top and bottom; underside of leaf is hairier. Leaf blades have bumps called floral nectaries. Flowers single, striking, to 5 inches in width.

Location: Worldwide distribution; numerous species found across seven climactic zones. Found wild in the southeast United States. Climbing vine of open areas and the forest edge. Most species tropical or subtropical, but will grow in a temperate garden. Often introduced.

Food: The leaf and flower tea has mild sedative properties. The fresh fruit may be eaten raw or juiced for a beverage. Mexicans mix passionflower blossoms and leaves with cornmeal or flour and eat

it as a gruel. Leaves are eaten by Native Americans. Typically leaves are parboiled and panfried in vegetable oil or animal fat.

Traditional uses: Fresh or dried aerial parts or the whole dried herb was used in infusion as a mild sedative as a sleep aid. Antispasmodic effect of the infusion was considered a gastrointestinal aid. People used the infusion of crushed root for treating earache. They also pounded the root and applied the mass as a poultice on inflamed contusions, boils, and cuts. The root water of the plant was mixed with lye-treated corn to wean babies. The tisane was considered a blood purifier for many tribes. Pioneers used the whole plant with Epsom salts as a sedative bath. Root tea and aerial parts tea were used for treating hemorrhoids.

Modern uses: Traditional uses are still employed. Commission E–approved for treating nervousness and insomnia. In animal studies the infusion was reported as sedative, antispasmodic, and inhibited

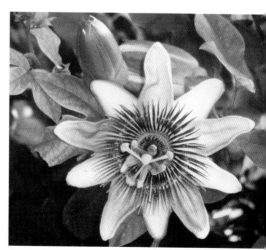

Passionflower, *Passiflora* sp.

motility of organisms. Its use as an antidepressive and for treating hysteria is unproven.

Notes: The Doctrine of Signatures suggests that this sensual-looking plant is an aphrodisiac. *Passiflora* has been found to contain beta-carboline harmala alkaloids that are monoamine oxidase inhibitors (MAOI) with antidepressant properties. Typically the flower has only traces of the chemicals, but the leaves and the roots of some species have been used to enhance the effects of mind-altering drugs.

Wildlife/veterinary uses: Fruit and seeds are of minor importance to birds. Several species are pollinated by hummingbirds, bumblebees, and wasps; still others are self-pollinating. *Passiflora* species are used as food plants by the larva of the moth *Cibyra serta* and by many Heliconiinae butterflies. The bracts of *P. foetida* are covered with hairs that exude a sticky fluid that traps insects. Studies have suggested that this may be an adaptation similar to that seen in carnivorous plants (Radhamani et al., *Journal of Biosciences*; see appendix D). *Passiflora* extract is used to calm stressed cats and has been used as a mild sedative for horses; see www .veterinarypracticenews.com.

Purslane
Portulaca oleracea L.

Description: Spreading, fleshy succulent annual that sprawls over the ground. Stems many branched, reddish. Leaves thick, fleshy, smooth and shiny, ovate or teardrop shaped (spatula shaped). Small, inconspicuous, yellowish flower in leaf rosettes. Blooms June through November.

Location: Nationwide. Gardens and waste ground.

Food: Purslane is a common garden plant, a volunteer alien creeper. It may be eaten right off the ground, put in salads, or chopped and added to soup. The payoff is omega-3 essential fatty acids. Native Americans ate the leaves as a raw or cooked vegetable. It was also boiled in soups and with meats. Try it chopped in salads, in salad dressing, even in turkey stuffing. Mexicans eat purslane raw with meat and green chilis or cooked with onions, carrots, beans, and chilis. Purslane can be dried and reconstituted as a winter food.

Traditional uses: Used as a poultice and a skin lotion. The whole plant in decoction was used to treat worms. Juice of the

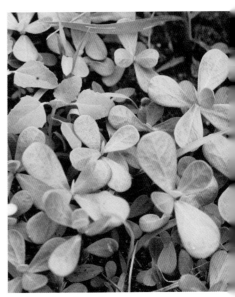

Purslane, *Portulaca oleracea*

whole plant considered a tonic and was also used to treat earaches. Purslane was an antidote to unspecified herbal toxins. Infusion of leaf stems was used to stem diarrhea. Mashed plant was applied as poultice over burns and bruises. Decoction of the whole plant was considered an antiseptic wash. Purslane was eaten to alleviate stomachache.

Modern uses: Purslane's essential fatty acids may help prevent inflammatory conditions such as heart disease, diabetes, and arthritis. Preparation extract is found in a few commercially available skin lotions.

Notes: I add the succulent leaves to salads and encourage this plant to grow in my garden. It is a natural and tasty way to get omega-3 fatty acids into my diet. If you won't eat it, add it to your mulch pile. The worms will prosper!

Wildlife/veterinary uses: In Mexico this is an important fodder for wildlife and domestic animals, especially free-range chickens, providing essential fatty acids.

Saint-John's-wort
Hypericum perforatum L.

Description: Stiff, almost woody stem, reddish and erect; may grow to 4 feet in height. Leaves ovate, attached at the base, and covered by glands. (Hold leaves toward the sun and you will see the glands; they appear as small perforations in the leaf.) Stems bear five-sepaled yellow flowers in terminal cymes (clusters). Sepals are marked with numerous glands. Blossoms have numerous stamens fused into three bundles. Cylindri-

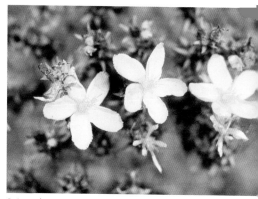

Saint-John's-wort, *Hypericum perforatum*

cal seeds are 1 to 3 millimeters long, black or brown, covered with small wart-like markings.

Location: Nationwide. Roadsides, waste ground, fields, prairies. There are numerous garden varieties.

Traditional uses: The whole-plant decoction was used to induce abortions by promoting menstruation. Parts used included the fresh and dried flowers, buds, and leaves. Topical applications rubbed on sores may have antiviral, antibacterial, and wound-healing activity. It was considered anti-inflammatory, antibacterial, antiviral, antidiarrheal, and astringent. Traditionally used for 2,000 years, initially in Greece to drive out evil spirits. Flower infusion or flower tincture was said to calm nerves, relieve insomnia, and boost mood by dispelling lethargy, like a nervine. Internally, tea was used as a PMS treatment. Tea, standardized capsule, and tincture were used to treat sciatica, anxiety, shingles, and fibrositis. Chewed root was considered a snakebite remedy. Crushed leaves and flowers were stuffed in nose to stem nosebleed.

Modern uses: Several studies in Europe show the benefit of this herb to treat mild depression. A standardized extract of 0.3 percent hypericin, 300 milligrams three times a day, was found comparable in antidepressant effect to a drug standard of imipramine. A recent study suggests a 5 percent hyperforin extract of the plant showed a slight increase in cognitive function. Other trials suggest that the drug may combat fatigue, relieve anxiety, improve sleep, help with weight loss, and attenuate menopausal symptoms. One study showed it relieved some forms of atopic dermatitis but was no more effective than placebo for treating major depression. It may work better than fluoxetine in treating depression (M. Fava et al., *Journal of Clinical Psychopharmacology; see appendix D).

An external infusion of flowers and leaves is used as a cooling, astringent, wound-healing infection fighter. It is antiviral and anti-inflammatory and is said to promote healing when used externally as a poultice or wash for infections, burns, bruises, sprains, tendonitis, sprains, neuralgia, or cramps. In vitro studies show a widespread antimicrobial activity against influenza, herpes simplex I and II, retrovirus, polio virus, sindbis virus, murine cytomegalovirus, hepatitis C, and gram negative and gram positive bacteria. It appears that exposure to ultraviolet light increases its antimicrobial activity.

Saint-John's-wort is available over the counter as a dietary supplement. Check with your health practitioner for appropriate use and dosage.

CAUTION: Not to be used to treat severe depression or bipolar depression. Extracts when used in German trials induced side effects in 2.4 percent of the test group. Side effects included gastrointestinal irritation, restlessness, and mild allergic reactions. It appears to be synergistic, with serotonin reuptake inhibitors, thereby increasing serotonin levels. Use of the supplement may lower activity of simultaneously administered drugs, including nonsedating antihistamines, oral contraceptives, certain antiretrovirals, antiepileptics, calcium channel blockers, cyclosporine, some chemotherapeutics, antibiotics, and select antifungals. Recent evidence suggests the chronic long-term use (abuse) of Saint-John's-wort is undesirable and may have negative health consequences. Purchase prepared products and only after consultation with your health-care professional.

Notes: I have used both a decoction and tincture of the whole plant to treat psoriasis with no success.

Wildlife/veterinary uses: Saint-John's-wort has been indicated in cattle poisoning. When consumed by livestock, the plant may also induce photosensitivity. For more information go to www.vet.purdue.edu and search for "plant toxins."

Heal-all, Self-heal
Prunella vulgaris L.

Description: Perennial typically 6 to 10 inches tall. Square stem erect when young; may fall and creep. Leaves ovate to lance shaped, margins dentate (toothed) to entire, and opposite. Blue to violet bract of flowers clustered in a whorl at end of square stem.

Location: Nationwide. Waste ground, lawns, edges of fields, margins of woods.

Food: According to Moerman (*Native American Ethonobotany;* see appendix D), the Cherokees cooked and ate small leaves. The Thompson First Peoples made a cold infusion of the aerial parts and drank this as a common beverage.

Traditional uses: Documented as used by the Chinese for more than 2,200 years, self-heal was used for liver complaints and improving the function of the liver. The whole plant was used in infusion to stimulate the liver and gallbladder and to promote healing. It is considered alterative; that is, capable of changing the course of a chronic disease.

Modern uses: Heal-all is still used internally by holistic practitioners to treat excessive menstruation and externally to treat burns, cuts, sores, and sore throats. The whole plant is infused and gargled for ulcers of the mouth and throat. The tea is made with 1 teaspoon of the dried

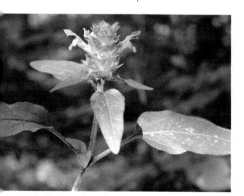

Heal-all, *Prunella vulgaris*

whole aerial parts of the plant to 1 cup of water as a remedy for diarrhea and unspecified gynecological disorders. Consult with a professional holistic healthcare professional for specific formulations and applications.

Notes: Locate this plant to your garden so you have it on-site and handy when you need it.

Wildlife/veterinary uses: Eaten by grazing animals.

Spiderwort, Widow's Tears, Spider Plant
Tradescantia virginiana L.; *T. occidentalis* (Britt.), Smyth; *T. pinetorum* Greene

Description: Perennial to 4 feet in height. Numerous leaves grow from the base (no stem). Leaves long, tough, swordlike, smooth; with entire margins. Flowers orchidlike, in drooping terminal clusters, deep blue; opening in morning and closing by afternoon. Blooms continuously through summer. There are at least four species in North America.

Location: Nationwide. Railroad right-of-ways, roadsides, fields, prairies, in my garden.

Food: Tender springtime shoots of *T. virginiana* and *T. occidentalis* are eaten raw or cooked. Flowers are edible throughout the year. Pick them in the morning before they wilt. Try them in salads or stir-fries or right off the plant. Flowers may be dipped in egg white and coated with powdered sugar.

Traditional uses: *T. virginiana* root tea was used as a laxative, to treat female kidney disorders, and for stomach problems. The aerial infusion was used to treat stomachache. Crushed and smashed aerial parts of the plant were applied as a poultice over insect bites and stings and used to bind wounds. Native Americans and pioneers used the crushed plant as a poultice to treat cancer. *T. occidentalis* tea was used as a diuretic. This plant infused is said to be an aphrodisiac.

Modern uses: Flowers have health-protecting flavonoids that may lower blood pressure (hypotensive), are diuretic, and may improve distal circulation. There is little or no modern evidence supporting the use of this medieval drug. The mucilaginous consistency of the young shoots, when eaten, may help alleviate sinus and bronchial spasms as well as soothe a sore throat (all unproven treatments).

Notes: Flowers open in morning, wilt by afternoon, and turn into a jellylike mass by evening. Hairy stamens of the flower have large rows of thin-walled cells in a chainlike

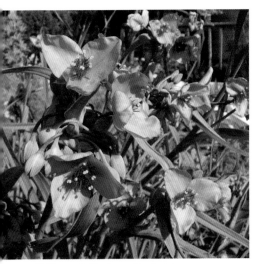

Spiderwort, *Tradescantia virginiana*

pattern. The flowing cytoplasm and nuclei of these cells can be easily seen under a microscope. The tough leaves of this plant can be used for binding wounds and woven into cordage. The Mixteca tribe of Mexico bound Cortez's thigh wound with this plant and are thus credited with saving his life. As a garden perennial this plant gives and gives and gives.

Wildlife/veterinary uses: *T. occidentalis* and *T. pinetorum* were fed to livestock to induce breeding (aphrodisiac). A cold infusion of the same plants were used to treat "deer infection" contracted from animals. Plant juice and strewn plants are said to be insect repellents.

Jimsonweed, Datura

Datura stramonium L.; *D. discolor* Bernh.

Description: Annual to 3 feet. Leaves toothed, coarse textured. Distinctive trumpetlike flower, white to light violet. Seed capsule studded with spines. Plant has musty odor.

Location: *D. stramonium* is found along roadsides and in bean and cornfields throughout the United States. *D. discolor*, more common in the Southwest and Four Corners area, has become a popular, showy garden flower throughout the Midwest.

Food: Not used as food; toxic.

Traditional uses: This plant is Native American Big Medicine. The whole plant and especially the seeds contain the alkaloids atropine and scopolamine. Atropine was used traditionally to dilate pupils. Leaves were smoked by Native Ameri-

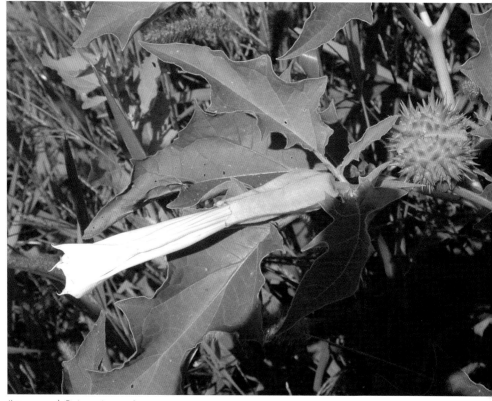

Jimsonweed, *Datura stramonium*

cans to treat asthma and other respiratory conditions. Smoking the leaves may also induce hallucinations. Numerous Indian nations used the plant as a ceremonial medicine. In a ritual that initiated young men into adulthood, datura roots were powdered and taken as a hallucinogen and narcotic purportedly to transform the user into a powerful animal. Powdered leaves were mixed with grease and used as an ointment, analgesic, and disinfectant. The whole plant was used symbolically to divine cures for disease and as a wash for cuts, wounds, and swellings. A paste of the plant was applied to insect bites, snake envenomations, and spider bites. Pioneers and folk practitioners used preparations of the seeds and leaves as an expectorant and to treat asthma, bronchitis, and flu.

Modern uses: Scopolamine is used in a popular motion sickness patch to treat dizziness and sea sickness. Scopolamine patches are used to treat asthma. Atropine is a sedative to the parasympathetic nerves and has been used in treating Parkinson's disease. Homeopathic practitioners use a preparation to treat cramps, eye inflammations, and infection. In China datura is still smoked to manage pain, treat asthma, and relieve arthritis.

CAUTION: Fatalities have been reported from abuse of this plant, typically from eating the seed. It is not to be used unless under the supervision of a professional health-care practitioner. According to Steven Foster and James Duke in *A Field Guide to Medicinal Plants: Eastern and Central North America*, licorice (*Glycyrrhiza*) may be an antidote to the toxic properties of the alkaloids in this plant.

Notes: I was called in to lecture at a local high school where a few students were abusing the drug. The lethal dose and the dose to get high are alarmingly close. All those spines on the seed capsules fairly scream: "Stay away from me!"

Wildlife/veterinary uses: Datura contamination of hay has caused extensive livestock poisoning. Dogs brought into contact with the plant have exhibited anisocoria (inequality in size of the pupils). All aerial parts of *D. stramonium* produced anisocoria following simple contact with the eye.

Comfrey
Symphytum officinale L.

Description: Perennial. Leaves start in spring from basal rosette of leaves from which grows stiff, erect stem to 4 feet or more. Leaves wrinkled and rough to the touch; basal leaves more ovate; upper leaves long, broadly lance shaped. Pale purple to violet flowers appear atop stem, arranged in crowded hanging cymes. Flowers have fused calyx with five tips and a fused five-tipped corolla with a pentangular tube.

Location: Rarely found outside the garden, at least by this author. Said to have

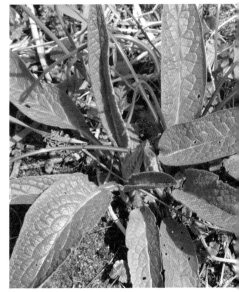

Comfrey, *Symphytum officinale*

escaped to waste ground and roadsides nationwide. Will grow in shade or full sun and is aggressive and spreading. Can be purchased at nurseries and from herb cottages.

Food: Leaves are made into tea and eaten by indigenous people worldwide. Comfrey is widely used in Japan, where it is cultivated and pickled. But it is not recommended as a food because research has shown the presence of liver-toxic pyrrolizidine alkaloids. Levels of pyrrolizidine alkaloids are highest in roots.

Traditional uses: External poultices were applied to bruises, swellings, sprains, and burns and to accelerate healing of broken bones. Leaf tea was used to treat ulcers, hemorrhoids, bronchitis, and congestion.

Modern uses: Comfrey extract is Commission E–approved for treating blunt injuries. It has scientifically proven anti-inflammatory action against rheumatism (the extract studied was a pyrrolizidine alkaloid–free product in an ointment; see M. Kucera et al., *Advanced Therapies,* in appendix D). Comfrey is a mucilaginous, cooling herb that contains allantoin. It appears to stimulate cell growth and is used in wound-healing skin creams. The leaf tea is still used under medical supervision to treat chronic bronchial problems, ulcers, colitis, arthritis, and rheumatism. Allantoin extracted from comfrey is available from your pharmacy; use it instead of the whole comfrey plant to avoid potential toxins.

CAUTION: Use of comfrey roots and leaves may cause cancer and destruction of the liver. Not recommended for use by lactating or pregnant women. Even external use of comfrey may cause assimilation of the toxic alkaloids.

Notes: An attractive and aggressive perennial garden dweller, this exotic-looking plant does well in temperate regions.

Wildlife/veterinary uses: A recent study showed that bees pollinating comfrey flowers carried toxic pyrrolizidine alkaloids to their hives and the substance was found in trace amounts in honey (*Science News* 161, no. 20 [2002]). Comfrey is an herbal constituent of Training Mix, a performance formulation for horses.

Wild Yam
Dioscorea villosa L.; *D. composita* Hemsl

Description: Sprawling, climbing perennial vine. Reddish brown stem may grow to 35 feet. Leaves typically alternate, broadly ovate to heart shaped; smooth on top, hairy underneath (pubescent). Flowers small, greenish yellow. Male flowers are drooping; female flowers are drooping and racemelike. The root and rhizome are used; rhizome is pale brown, a twisted tuberous cylinder.

Location: Canada to the southern United States. Tropical, subtropical, and temperate conditions.

Food: Wild yams are used in Chinese medicinal soups and sold in Chinese supermarkets and Chinese drugstores. Add about 20 grams of the sliced, dried root to chicken stock; simmer; add vegetables, meat, and garlic . . . serve. The tubers are bitter and considered toxic, but Chinese uses challenge that contention. Be careful.

Traditional uses: Meskwaki Indians used the decoction of the root as an analgesic

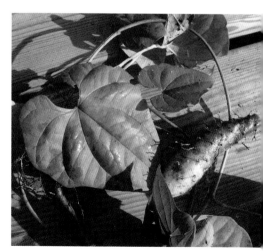

Wild yam, *Dioscorea* sp.

for birthing and postpartem pain. Dried wild yam root slices are taken with Solomon's seal (*Polygonatum*) root to treat dysmenorrhea in traditional Chinese medicine. Indigenous people of South America traditionally used the root to treat pain of menstruation and labor (ovarian pain). Also used for arthritis, as a digestive aid, and for muscle cramping. Considered to have anti-inflammatory, antispasmodic, antiarthritic, warming, and diuretic properties.

Modern uses: Diosgenin from wild yam (a breakdown component of dioscin) was the model material for the birth control pill. DHEA and other hormones and hormone-starter materials are fabricated from the phytosterols in the root of wild yam. Japanese scientists developed corticosteroid compounds from the root-starter material. Tea is occasionally prescribed by naturopaths for irritable bowel syndrome, and a tincture may be prescribed for arthritis. Root decoctions are taken for chronic fatigue, nocturnal emissions, neurasthenia (similar to chronic fatigue), insomnia, neurosis, and feelings of inadequacy. The chopped root can be made into tea or tinctured in 30 to 40 percent alcohol; see Chevallier, *Encyclopedia of Medicinal Plants* (appendix D) for information. A commercially prepared drug from wild yam is taken for leukorrhea, a whitish, viscid vaginal discharge. As a poultice the smashed root is applied to abscesses, boils, and skin sores.

CAUTION: Not to be taken internally by people with high blood pressure or constipation. Check with your holistic health-care practitioner. Do not take wild yam during pregnancy without a physician's guidance.

Notes: Once started in your garden, wild yam is difficult to eradicate—it will raise its pretty head here, there, and everywhere. Grown along a wall or fence, it makes an unusually attractive cover.

Wildlife/veterinary uses: Wild yam is part of an herbal treatment for horses (see www.racehorseherbal.com). The root extract is said to help in treating senility in animals and central nervous system problems. DHEA extracted from wild yam doubled the life of rats.

Baptisia, False Indigo

Baptisia australis (L.) R. Br. ex Ait. f.; *B. tinctoria* L.

Description: Tall, shrublike perennial to 5 feet in height. Pealike leaves. Striking blue, pealike flowers. Clusters of large indigo seedpods. *B. tinctoria* has clover-like leaves, yellow blooms.

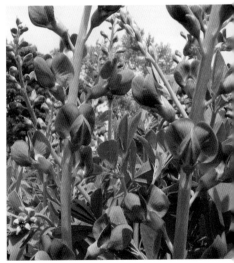

Baptisia, *Baptisia australis*

Location: Prairie wildflower both east and west of the Mississippi. Garden ornamental.

Food: Not edible.

Traditional uses: Native Americans used a decoction of the roots to treat wounds, bites, and stings. Considered an immune-stimulating herb used in decoction as a vaginal douche for vaginitis. A poultice of the root was applied over venereal disease sores. A cold infusion of the smashed root was a purgative and emetic. The root infusion was used to wash wounds.

Modern uses: The root extract is considered a fair infection fighter when used in the hands of a skilled medical practitioner. Toxic dose will cause nausea and vomiting. The homeopathic dose is considered safe and is said to improve immune defense mechanisms by raising leukocyte counts (see *PDR for Herbal Medicines,* third edition). Animal studies showed the polysaccharide fraction stimulates the immune system.

CAUTION: Taken orally, the root decoction is potent and toxic.

Notes: My daughter uses the ripe seedpods and seeds in a sun tea infusion to extract a blue dye. False indigo is a striking, decorative plant in the perennial garden. Flowers and seedpod stalks are attractive additions to flower arrangements.

Wildlife/veterinary uses: This shrubby plant provides storm shelter and refuge for small songbirds and is a host plant for insects and butterflies. Without endorsing it, I mention Phyto-Biotic, a botanical antimicrobial product containing *B. tinctoria* root bark, *Allium sativum* bulb, *Echinacea angustifolia* root, *Hydrastis canadensis* root, *Berberis vulgaris* root, and *Phytolacca americana* root.

California Poppy
Eschscholzia californica Cham.

Description: Annual or perennial, 15 to 40 inches tall. Leaves few, bluish green, tapering to a point, feathery or fernlike. Brilliant yellow orange solitary flowers. Cup- or bowl-shaped seed receptacle contains several chambers filled with tiny seeds. Hundreds of species.

Location: California to British Columbia. Open areas, roadsides, dry clearings. Also in gardens nationwide.

Food: Native Americans of the Luiseno Nation ate young springtime leaves as cooked greens. The leaves were first boiled, then fried or roasted and eaten. Poppy seeds may be purchased over the counter.

Traditional uses: Aerial parts are harvested, dried, and infused as a sleep-inducing sedative. It has been used for anxiety, for nervousness, and as an antispasmolytic. It is considered a warming agent and a diuretic and has an analgesic effect. Folk use includes treating nocturnal urinating in children. Native Americans used the milky sap of the leaves as an analgesic to relieve toothaches. Leaves were also placed under children at bedtime to induce sleep. The white resin from seedpods was rubbed on a nursing mother's breast to promote lactation.

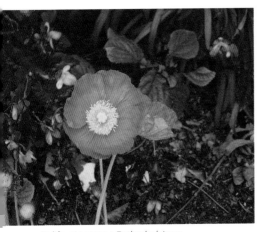

California poppy, *Eschscholzia* sp.

However, several tribes believed the plant to be poisonous and avoided its use.

Modern uses: Californidine, an alkaloid in the plant, is used as a sleep aid and sedative. These qualities have been proven in animal studies only. Homeopathic preparations are used to treat insomnia.

CAUTION: Not to be used during pregnancy or by nursing mothers.

Notes: This attractive, deep-rooted, spreading addition to your garden provides edible seeds.

Wildlife/veterinary uses: A food source for small mammals and terrestrial birds. In California it is illegal to pick this plant, as it is the state flower.

Flax, Linseed
Linum usitatissimum L.

Description: Delicate-looking annual to 3 feet in height. Gray green leaves lance shaped, smooth edged. Sky blue flowers born in leaf axils on upper part of slender stem. Flowers have five sepals and five ovate petals with five stamens and one ovary. Seeds flat, brown, glossy.

Location: Temperate-zone plant. Roadsides, barns, waste ground near where the plant has escaped cultivation. Buy flaxseeds at a health-food store and spread them in your garden.

Food: Mix flaxseeds in salads, waffles, or pancakes; blend them into juice drinks; or eat them whole out of hand. Tip: Grind seeds before adding them to juice, cereal, and other foods to release the oils. They are healthful in bread and corn bread—in all baking, in fact—and are especially beneficial when used uncooked or very lightly cooked. See the video *Diet for Natural Health* (appendix D) for numerous recipes using flax and other essential dietary fats. Flax flowers are edible.

Traditional uses: The Greeks and Romans considered flax a panacea. Native Americans used flax as food and medicine to treat inflammatory diseases and infections: colds, coughs, fevers, and painful urination. These early uses suggested the now-known anti-inflammatory effect of flax.

Modern uses: Flaxseed is one of the highest plant sources of omega-3 fatty acids. (Perilla seeds at your Oriental grocery contain slightly more omega-3.) This essential fatty acid is a memory and cognitive-mind enhancer. Omega-3s protect us from degenerative diseases. Increasing the ratio of omega-3 to omega-6 in the American diet may

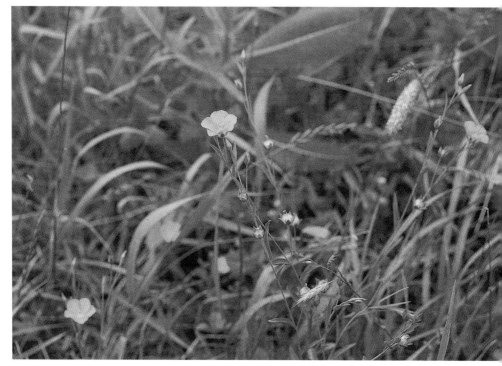

Flax, *Linum usitatissimum*

prevent more autoimmune and inflammatory diseases. The husk of the seed has lignins, mucilage, and phenolics that provide extra protection from heart disease, cancer, and diabetes.

Flax is Commission E–approved for treating inflammations of the skin and constipation. Clinical trials have shown the efficacy of the supplement (oil) to lower cholesterol and raise plasma levels of insulin. As an antiplatelet aggregating agent, it may decrease the potential for thrombosis.

Notes: I was told by a medical doctor that not all folks convert the omega fats from flaxseeds into omega-3 fatty acids as efficiently as others. He suggested eating cold-water fish—salmon, herring, sardines, and mackerel—or taking fish-oil supplements as the preferred sources of the vital-to-life essential fats. I take the advice with a grain of salt, as the same physician sells a line of fish-oil supplements.

Wildlife/veterinary uses: Flaxseed is a vital component of premium wild and domestic bird feeds and food mixes for racing animals like horses, birds, and dogs. Flaxseed is also used in veterinarian medicine in the United States, Europe, and India. It's an integral part of Power Dust wound treatment for horses.

CHAPTER 2

Medicinal Herbs of Eastern Forested Areas

The Great Spirit above has appointed this place for us, on which to light our fires, and here we will remain.

—TECUMSEH

The following medicinal plants are found in forested areas of the United States. Bear in mind that biomes often overlap, and you may discover these plants in areas of transition—from field to forest, for example, or the transition zone from forest to marsh or along wood-lined roadsides.

Skunk Cabbage
Symplocarpus foetidus (L.) Nutt.

Description: Large, green, elephant ear–like leaves, lustrous and waxy in appearance, with skunky odor when torn. Flower is archaic, showy spathelike sheathing surrounding a clublike spadix.

Location: Eastern United States. Wet woods, swamps, lowlands, wet coastal areas. (The western skunk cabbage, *Lysichiton americanus,* is found west of the Rockies.)

Food: The eastern species is little used as food.

Traditional uses: The liquid extract was used to treat bronchitis and asthma. Native Americans dried the root of the eastern species and used it as antispasmodic tea to stop seizures (epilepsy), coughs, asthma, or toothache. A paste of dried root was used externally for skin irritations to quell itching. A crushed-leaf poultice was used externally on swellings and as an analgesic and was considered antirheumatic. The dried-root infusion

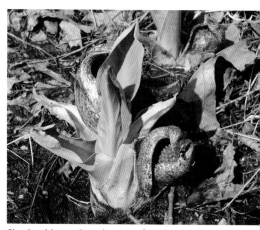

Skunk cabbage, *Symplocarpus foetidus*

was used to treat coughs and the root also was applied as a poultice over wounds. A decoction of crushed stalks served as a douche to improved displacement of the womb. Leaves were chewed to treat epilepsy. The dried, powdered root was given as infusion to treat convulsions.

Modern uses: A liquid extract of skunk cabbage is still used to treat bronchitis and asthma. The plant is considered antispasmodic, expectorant, sedative, and diaphoretic. Its use is reserved for skilled practitioners only.

CAUTION: Skunk cabbage contains poisonous oxalate crystals. Juice from the fresh plant may cause skin blistering and will severely burn the digestive tract if eaten. Only experts should handle this plant. Although its name suggests that it is edible, it requires exhaustive preparation in several changes of water to yield mediocre results.

Notes: I have eaten the raw leaf of the eastern species and regretted it. It tasted as if a gnome had pounded a thousand needles in my tongue. Avoid using the fresh parts of this plant as food or medicine.

Wildlife/veterinary uses: Botanically, skunk cabbage is endothermic: It actually produces heat that often melts snow and ice around its base. Thus it is one of the earliest-flowering plants of spring.

Hepatica, American Liverwort

Hepatica nobilis var. *obtusa* (Pursh) Steyermark (also known as *H. triloba* and *H. americana*); *H. nobilis* var. *acuta* (Pursh) Steyermark (also known as *H. acutiloba*)

Description: Small perennial to 5 inches in height. Leaves basal, evergreen, with the difference between the two species determined by the end shape of their leaves: rounded vs. pointed. *H. nobilis* var. *acuta* is sharp lobed; *H. nobilis* var. *obtusa* is round lobed. Stems and leaves are hairy when they emerge. Flowers of *H.* var. *acuta* are violet to blue, and *H.* var. *obtusa* has whitish blossoms all with six to ten sepals. American liverwort is one of the first spring flowers, blooming in March or April.

Location: Eastern forests west to Nebraska and north into Canada.

Traditional uses: Native Americans infused *H. nobilis* var. obtusa and used it as an emetic, laxative, and abortifacient.

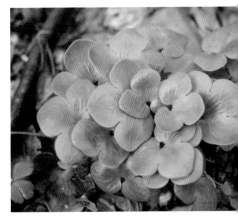

Hepatica, *Hepatica nobilis* var. *obtusa*

As an infusion *H.* var. *obtusa* was considered contraceptive. The Menominees used leaf infusions and root decoctions to treat diarrhea and vertigo. Because the leaves look like lobes of the liver, the leaf tea was used to treat liver problems (in accordance with the Doctrine of Signatures, or "like treats like"). Folk practitioners used small amounts of the roots and leaves of hepatica to treat indigestion and disorders of the kidney, gallbladder, and liver. Sharp-lobed hepatica (*H. nobilis* var. *acuta*) was used in decoction as aid to digestion and with pregnant women to ease labor pain. It was considered a tonic (a blood purifier). The decoction was used as a uterine stimulate to induce childbirth. The infusion was used to treat pain in the abdomen and as an emetic and laxative.

Modern uses: European practitioners still use the plant chemistry internally for liver disorders, including gallstones.

CAUTION: Large amounts of hepatica are poisonous. Use it only under the supervision of a professional holistic medical practitioner.

Notes: Look, enjoy, but don't eat or touch hepatica: External contact with the plant can cause dermatitis, and internally it is caustic to the intestinal tract and the urinary plumbing.

Wildlife/veterinary uses: Native Americans and pioneers spread a decoction of hepatica on snares, traps, or guns to lure furbearing animals.

Bloodroot, Red Puccoon, Red Indian Paint

Sanguinaria canadensis L.

Description: Perennial to 7 inches in height. Rhizome thick and slightly curved; exudes red liquid when cut; rootlets are reddish. Leaves down covered, grayish green, and clasping; growing in a basal rosette, with five to nine lobes, accented underneath with protruding rips. Flower is single, white, with eight to twelve petals; short-lived, early spring bloomer.

Location: Eastern forests south to Florida, west to Minnesota, and north to Manitoba. Damp, rich forests, along forest trails.

Food: Not edible.

Traditional uses: The extract from this toxic plant is antispasmodic and warming. Native Americans discovered that the herb induced vomiting. Pioneers and First Peoples used the root extraction in cough medicines and to treat rheumatism, fevers, and laryngitis. Some folk practitioners suggest that a very small dose works as an appetite stimulant. This may be attributed to the bitter alkaloids that stimulate the digestive system reflexively. The root juice was reportedly used to treat warts. It is anesthetic. Other reported uses were for treating bronchitis, throat infections, asthma, and other lung ailments.

Modern uses: Research shows that sanguinarine and chelerythrine found in bloodroot have anticancer properties. Cancer of nose and ear has responded to topical applications of bloodroot extract root and cancer in dogs. In veterinary medicine the leaf of bloodroot is used to destroy bot-fly larvae on horses.

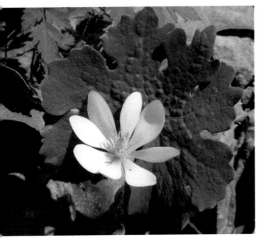

Bloodroot, *Sanguinaria canadensis*

in research trials. It is still used topically as an anti-inflammatory. Sanguinarine, although toxic, has low oral toxicity and is antiseptic. Small amounts of it are used in a name-brand mouthwash and tooth-paste.

CAUTION: Mildly toxic. Because of the plant's potential toxicity, it is little used as an expectorant in modern uses.

Notes: There are reports that the red bloodroot exudant, when thinned with water and applied to the skin, was an effective mosquito repellent. In tests on human beings, I have found this to be true. Perhaps the red skin of Native Americans observed by the invading Europeans was actually bloodroot applied as a mosquito repellent. The effect of long-term exposure of sanguinarine to the skin is unknown. To learn how I use the root juice to ward off mosquitoes, see the DVDs *Native American Medicine* and *Little Medicine* (appendix D).

Wildlife/veterinary uses: Visit www.dog cancer.com to read a discussion of blood-

Mayapple, American Mandrake
Podophyllum peltatum L.

Description: Perennial. Umbrella-like plant with cleft leaves. Two leaves on single, stout stalk, each leaf with five to seven lobes. Single white flower tucked under leaf. Fruit ripens from mid- to late summer; edible only when ripe. Plant colonies spread over the forest floor.

Location: Eastern forest dweller. Rich woods.

Food: The fruit may be eaten in summer when it is soft and ripe. The fruit is difficult to find: Many plants die off in summer, the plants do not always provide abundant fruit, and you are competing with forest creatures for the "apple." Cook the fruit or, if it is completely ripe, eat it out of hand. Use ripe fruit in pies, muffins, waffles, and pancakes or make it into jam or jelly. Native Americans smashed and dried the fruit as fruit cakes that were later reconstituted in water and used as a sauce.

Traditional uses: Minute doses of mayapple were used by Native Americans to treat a variety of illnesses. It treated verrucae (warts produced by papillomavirus). It is an emetic and purgative—a powerful laxative. The root is toxic and was used to kill worm infestations. Root powder was applied externally on difficult-to-heal sores. Fresh juice from the root (approximately 1 drop) was put in the ear to improve hearing. It is said that a potent extract from mayapple was used by Native Americans to commit suicide. In the mid-twentieth century, mayapple resin was injected into venereal warts as a treatment.

Modern uses: *P. peltatum* is Commission E–approved for treating warts, specifically genital warts. The root extract contains an antimitotic agent that led to the formulation of synthetic etoposide, a treatment for small-cell lung cancer and testicular cancer. The roots and leaves are poisonous, and handling the roots may cause allergic dermatitis. Himalayan mayapple (*P. emodi*) is most rich in the toxic drug podophyllotoxin.

CAUTION: Avoid using this plant as a drug without medical supervision. The drug may be absorbed through the skin. It is an allergen, toxic, and antimitotic.

Notes: Mayapple is a showy ground cover most evident in spring, appearing about the same time I'm plucking morels. I prepare mayapple root water as an insecticide for my garden. Blend about 8

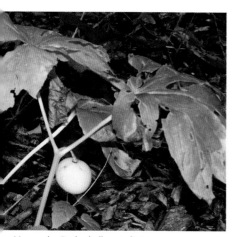

Mayapple, *Podophyllum peltatum*

ounces of fresh root in 2 quarts of water, then strain the mixture through cheesecloth or pantyhose into a garden sprayer. (For details about this procedure and many others, see the DVDs *Native American Medicine* and *Little Medicine;* appendix D.)

Wildlife/veterinary uses: The Menominees used an infusion of the crushed plant to kill potato bugs. Corn seeds and corn roots were soaked in a mayapple decoction to discourage fungus and other pests (see my notes above).

Jack-in-the-pulpit
Arisaema triphyllum (L.) Schott

Description: A 2-foot perennial with one or two leaves with three leaflets each. Spathe cuplike, with covering flap, green to purplish brown, striped, with scarlet berries in a cluster.

Location: Eastern United States. Moist forests, rich soils.

Food: The fruit of jack-in-the-pulpit is not edible. Indians sliced jack-in-the-pulpit roots and dried them, a process that is said to deactivate the caustic calcium oxalate. The dried root slices were then cooked and eaten like potato chips.

Traditional uses: The dried root was used to treat respiratory problems: asthma, bronchitis, colds, cough, and laryngitis. The externally poulticed root was used as wash for ringworm, sores, boils, and abscesses. Iroquois women reportedly used the root of *A. triphyllum* ssp. *triphyllum* in infusion as a contraceptive for temporary sterility.

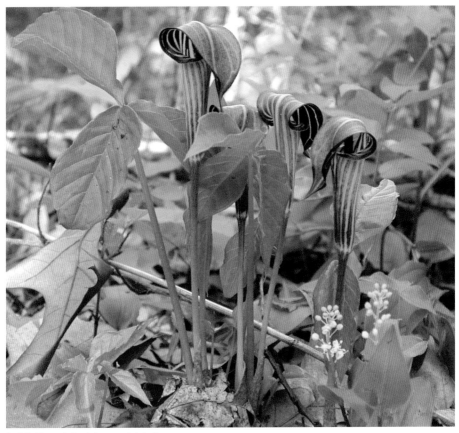

Jack-in-the-pulpit, *Arisaema triphyllum*

Modern uses: Members of the genus are still used to treat snakebite in western China.

CAUTION: Do not eat the fresh plant. It contains caustic oxalates when fresh and must be thoroughly dried before use. Handle with care: Calcium oxalate will cause painful burns in cracked skin or open sores.

Notes: Jack-in-the-pulpit transplants to a shaded, rich-soiled garden.

Wildlife/veterinary uses: If your pets ingest this plant, they may experience severe gastric distress. Iroquois peoples used the plant as a veterinary aid. They ground the plant and then added it to mare's feed to induce pregnancy and reduce listlessness.

Uva-ursi, Kinnikinnick, Bearberry
Arctostaphylos uva-ursi (L.) Spreng

Description: Trailing shrub, prostrate and mat forming. Leaves dark, evergreen, leathery, smooth edged, obovate or spatula shaped, less than ¾ inch wide. Alpine variety of bearberry has larger leaves. Fruit is a dry red berry.

Location: Northern United States and Canada.

Food: The berries are dry and mealy and lack flavor, so they were traditionally cooked with animal fat or mixed with fish eggs (such as salmon eggs) and stronger-tasting foods. Berries may be dried and then smashed into a flourlike meal. First Peoples of the Northwest used this flour like a spice with meat and organ meats. People of the Bella Coola Nation mixed berries in fat and ate them; Lower Chinook peoples dried the berries and then mixed them with fat for food. Many Native Americans boiled the berries with roots and vegetables to make a soup. You can sauté the berries in grease until crisp, then place them in cheesecloth or pantyhose and pound them to a mash. Add the mash to cooked fish eggs and stir, pound in some more mash and eggs, mix, then sweeten to taste.

Traditional uses: The whole plant was infused in water and mixed with grease from a goose, duck, bear, or mountain goat. Then glue cooked from an animal's hoof, either horse or deer, was mixed into the grease. The resulting salve was used on sores, babies' scalps, and rashes. An infusion of aerial parts was gargled as a mouthwash to treat canker sores and sore gums. Dried leaves and stems were ground and used as a poultice over wounds. An infusion of leaves, berries, and stems was taken orally for cleaning kidneys and bladder complaints as a diuretic. The same beverage had an analgesic effect on back pain and sprains. Berries were eaten or infused with whole plant for colds. Kwakiutl peoples smoked the leaves for the reported narcotic effect. Dried leaves were crushed to a powder and sprinkled on sores. Leaves and tobacco were mixed and placed in religious bundles for spiritual healing. Pioneers used the leaf infusion as a diuretic, astringent, and tonic.

Modern uses: Commission E–approved to treat infections of the urinary tract. It is commercially available dried, powdered in capsules, and as whole leaves for tea. There are numerous homeopathic preparations. The hot tea is considered styptic, astringent, and antibacterial. The tea as a diuretic increases urine flow. Also the tea internally and externally is considered antimicrobial and anti-inflammatory, and it has prevented kidney stone formation in lab animals.

CAUTION: Do not use during pregnancy or while nursing. Avoid eating acidic foods when using the tea to treat urogenital and biliary tract diseases. Prolonged use of uva-ursi may damage the liver and inflame and irritate the bladder and kidneys. Its use is not recommended for children.

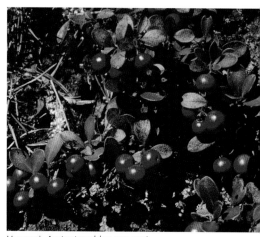

Uva-ursi, *Arctostapyhlos uva-ursi*

Notes: I've boiled the berries to make a grayish brown dye. Native Americans used an application of crushed berries to waterproof baskets.

Wildlife/veterinary uses: Several herbal formulas for horses incorporate uva-ursi, including formulas for joint rebuilding, protecting supplements, training mixes, and fertility boosters.

Wintergreen, Teaberry, Checkerberry, Canada Tea
Gaultheria procumbens L.

Description: Small evergreen to 5 or 6 inches in height, often shorter in dry woods. Spreads by adventitious roots. Leaves evergreen, oval, growing on the tips of the branches; glossy above, paler underneath. Flowers white, waxy, drooping bells. Fruit is pale white berry, red when ripe.

Location: Northern United States and Canada. Forest dweller, typically subarboreal but found spreading in open areas of woods.

Food: This plant makes a pleasant wintergreen tea. I prefer to chew on the fresh leaf while walking in woods. My two favorite chew sticks are wintergreen and sassafras. The berries are scarce and bland but fun to look for. The leaf tea, leaf chew, and berries are the safest way to experience the unusual flavor of this plant. The dried-leaf tea has a different taste than fresh leaf tea—try it both ways. Wintergreen is a flavoring for gum and an aromatic in candle making. The oils of clove, sassafras, and wintergreen have been made into beverages. The tea is used as a gargle for sore throat relief.

Traditional uses: The plant was considered anodyne; astringent; diuretic; stimulant; emmenagoge; lactagogue. Leaf tea was used to treat stomachaches, fevers, colds, headaches, kidney ailments, and dysmenorrhea (avoid drinking wintergreen tea during pregnancy). The tea was used externally as a wash reportedly to ease rheumatism and muscle aches. Native Americans roasted (dried) the leaves and smoked them with tobacco.

Modern uses: Wintergreen oil is little used today, occasionally in ointments and liniments to treat neuralgia or sciatica. Wintergreen oil is antiseptic and astringent.

CAUTION: Overuse of the herb must be avoided. Fatalities have occurred taking oral and subcutaneous doses of the essential oil. Amounts of 4 grams have been toxic and fatal. The oil has caused allergic reactions. Do not use wintergreen oil or tea during pregnancy.

Notes: Wintergreen leaves are a pleasant chew on long hikes. It's a sialagogue—a

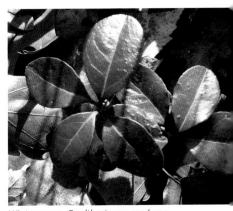

Wintergreen, *Gaultheria procumbens*

substance that increases the production of saliva and thus brings moisture to the mouth.

Wildlife/veterinary uses: Berries are eaten by chipmunk, deer, grouse, and partridge; leaves are browse for deer and moose. Wintergreen oil is one of several essential oils in a patent described as a method for increasing bioavailability of an orally administered hydrophobic pharmaceutical compound that is to be absorbed in the gut to treat animals. A Tigerbalm-like oil that contains wintergreen, camphor, eucalyptus, lavender, peppermint, and almond oil is available for use with your pets. For the recipe visit the Veterinary Botanical Medicine Association Web site, www.vbma.org, then search "peppermint."

Lady's Slipper Orchid
Cypripedium acaule Aiton

Description: Perennial. Leaves lilylike, basal, stalkless, broadly lance shaped, to 10 inches in length, bright green above and pale underneath. Horizontal rhizome gives rise to orchidlike, slipper-shaped flower, typically pink, rarely white. Fruit capsule brown.

Location: Northern United States and Canada. Upland pine forests, wet black spruce sites. Occasionally open wetlands. More prolific in the northeastern states and southern Ontario. Grows in profusion along the north shore of Lake Superior.

Food: Not eaten.

Traditional uses: The horizontal rhizome (root) contains the active principle. It is styptic and astringent, considered a

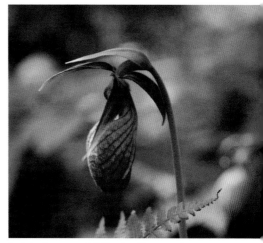

Lady's slipper orchid, *Cypripedium acaule*

superior nervine (tranquilizer) and therefore overharvested in the wild. The rhizome was used in decoction or tincture and considered by Native Americans as a panacea for nervousness, colds, cramps, diabetes, flu, hysteria, menstrual problems, spasms, and inflammations (applied as a poultice). The rhizome is harvested in autumn and used fresh or dried for later use. Following the Doctrine of Signatures, this plant was once considered one of nature's finest aphrodisiacs because of the flower's shape.

Modern uses: This plant has been overharvested and is now protected, so its legal use has been discontinued. Its chemical constituents have not been tested.

CAUTION: Contact with pink lady's slipper may cause contact dermatitis.

Notes: During Memorial Day weekend, Lake Superior Provincial Park on Lake Superior is ablaze with pink lady's slippers. Bring your kayak. There are a dozen lady's slipper–studded islands just a stone's throw offshore. The species is widely protected from illegal harvesting.

Wildlife/veterinary uses: Lady's slippers are difficult to relocate because of a complex symbiosis with soil fungi. Bees, moths, butterflies, gnats, and mosquitoes pollinate the orchids.

Black Cohosh
Actaea racemosa (L.) Nutt.

Description: Perennial to 5½ feet in height. Rhizome, blackish, knotty, tough. Leaves double pinnate, smooth, serrated. Flower raceme drooping, with three to eight petals. Sepals enclose flower bud.

Location: Northern United States and southern Canada. Forests.

Food: Not a food.

Traditional uses: The root (rhizome) is the medicinal part. Root infusions were used to induce abortions, stimulate menstruation, and promote lactation. An alcohol infusion of the root was used to treat rheumatism. The infused root was taken to treat coughs and was said to be cathartic and stimulating, a tonic and blood purifier. Pulverized roots in hot bathwater were used as a soak to alleviate arthritis pain.

Modern uses: The plant extract is Commission E–approved for premenstrual syndrome and menopausal complaints. Commercial preparations are used to treat female conditions including uterine spasms (cramps), menstrual pain, hot flashes, mild depression, vaginal atrophy, and menopause. The estrogenic effect reduces luteinizing hormone levels. A recent study of the use of Remifemin, a proprietary black cohosh extraction, significantly reduced hot flashes, and psyche disturbances in a trial group from 304 postmenopausal women (Friede, Liske, et al., *Obstetric Gynecology* 105 [2005]: 1074–83). The study results confirmed the efficacy and tolerability of an isopropanolic extract of black cohosh. Forty-six percent of breast cancer survivors who received a black cohosh preparation were symptom free of hot flashes, sweating, and other symptoms of anxiety and sleep disturbances related to premenopausal breast cancer treatment (Jacobson, *Journal of Clinical Oncology* 19, no. 10 [2001]: 2739–45). And a 2003 study showed an increase of bone formation in postmenopausal women (Wuttke et al., *Maturitas* 44 [2003]: S67–S77). Holistic health practitioners still use the plant for treating fever, arthritis, and insomnia.

CAUTION: Consult a licensed holistic health-care practitioner before using this herb for dysmenorrhea, hormone replacement therapy, or menopausal

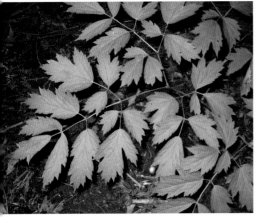

Black cohosh, *Actaea racemosa*

symptoms. Avoid completely if you are lactating or pregnant.

Notes: The United Kingdom health-care products regulatory agency (MHRA) and the European Medicines Agency (EMEA) have warned patients to stop using black cohosh if they develop signs suggestive of liver toxicity (blood in urine, tiredness, loss of appetite, yellowing of skin or eyes, stomach pain, nausea, vomiting, or dark urine). In the United Kingdom a warning must appear on the label of black cohosh products. For details visit www.herbal gram.org and search "black cohosh regulations."

Wildlife/veterinary uses: Black cohosh is used in a proprietary horse product called Fertility Boost.

Blue Cohosh, Squaw Root, Papoose Root

Caulophyllum thalictroides (L.) Michx.

Description: Leafy perennial to 30 inches in height. Grows erect from a brown gray, branched rhizome. Leaves tripinnate; leaflets stemmed, ovate, finely divided, with three lobes, wedge shaped at the base. Flowers arise from terminal leaf; yellowish green to purple flowers, about ½ inch wide, with six sepals arranged in two rows and six inconspicuous petals per flower. The ovary contains two dark blue roundish seeds about ⅛ inch in diameter.

Location: East from the Atlantic coast south to South Carolina and Arkansas, west including Minnesota and Iowa, and north to Canada. Wet woods.

Food: Not edible.

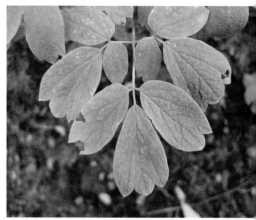
Blue cohosh, *Caulophyllum thalictroides*

Traditional uses: Used by Native Americans and in ethnic black medicine to ease and facilitate childbirth. It is claimed to have an analgesic and diuretic effect. Cherokees took the extract internally as an anticonvulsive and antirheumatic and crushed and rubbed leaves on poison oak and poison ivy. Chippewas scraped and decocted the root "skin" and used it as an emetic. The analgesic effect of the root decoction was said to take the edge off uterine cramps and nonspecific stomach cramps. Several tribes used the plant extract to stem profuse menstruation. It was also used as a sedative to settle "fits and hysterics." The Meskwakis and Mohegans used the herb to treat kidney and urinary problems.

Modern uses: Roots (rhizome) are prepared as a liquid extract to treat gynecological disorders. The extract appears to have an estrogenic effect and is used internally to treat dysmenorrhea, potential miscarriage, and uterine spasms. Homeopathic preparations are prescribed by health-care professionals. The Chinese use the drug for treating external

61

injuries and internally to treat bronchitis and acute hepatitis.

CAUTION: Because of the drug's heart- and uterine-stimulating effects, use of this plant is not recommended.

Notes: Like all unproven (and proven) remedies, use blue cohosh only under the skilled hands of a holistic health-care professional. Never take this uterine-stimulant during pregnancy or if you have hypertension or heart disease.

Wildlife/veterinary uses: The drug has a folk history as an abortifacient, but there is scant evidence it has induced abortions in animals.

Black Nightshade
Solanum nigrum L.

Description: Perennial to 30 inches in height. Erect stem with many branches with many leaves. Leaves fleshy, round to ovate, smooth to slightly hairy. White flowers bloom in the fall from umbel-like nodding group, six to ten blossoms. Each flower has five stamens. Fruit is pea-sized black (occasionally green to yellow) berry.

Location: Worldwide. Roadsides, fields, forest edges, waste ground.

Food: Cherokees ate the young plant cooked as a potherb. Fruit and berries were eaten and made into preserves and pies. Numerous plants of the nightshade family (Solanacea) are considered toxic; others are quite edible, such as potatoes, tomatoes, tomatillas, and peppers. Seek professional guidance before eating unknown species.

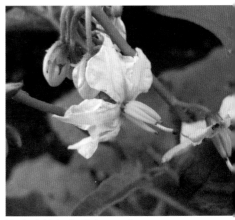

Black nightshade, *Solanum nigrum*

Traditional uses: The berry juice was used to treat tumors. The berries are diuretic. The plant juice was a laxative and an emollient. This solanaceous plant was used by Native Americans as an emetic. They applied it externally in decoction as a wash or poultice for skin ailments such as psoriasis, hemorrhoids, and eczema. Smoke of the dried plant was inhaled to treat toothache.

Modern uses: Ayurvedic practitioners consider the berries an aphrodisiac and tonic. Black nightshade is available dried and cut, powdered, and in liquid extracts. The moistened plant is used externally as a compress or rinse. Internal use should be carefully monitored by a holistic health-care professional. Plant extracts are used in Chinese and ayurvedic medicine both internally and externally. In India the plant is considered a panacea and used as a laxative and a tonic and to treat asthma, bronchitis, dysentery fever, heart disease, congestive heart failure, hiccups, and inflammation. The dried fruit powder is used as alterative, tonic, and diuretic.

Notes: There are several hybridized garden varieties of this herb. Hybridization not only changes the physical appearances of a plant, but it also affects its chemistry. A wild strain or hybrid of this plant should only be used under the supervision of a licensed holistic healthcare provider.

Wildlife/veterinary uses: Cattle, chickens, duck, horses, sheep, and swine have been poisoned eating the plant, according to James Duke (*Handbook of Medicinal Herbs;* see appendix D).

Ginseng

Panax ginseng C.A. Meyer; *P. quinquefolius* L.

Description: Perennial to 3 feet in height. Stem smooth, round. Three to five leaves in terminal whorls with three to five palmate leaflets; leaflets, finely serrated, 3 to 8 inches long, 1 to 2 inches wide. Greenish, yellow flowers give rise to a pea-sized, rounded, glossy seed.

Location: Cultivated from coast to coast, found wild in the Northwest and eastern forested areas. Rare in most of its former range. Needs shading forest with mature canopy and well-drained soil.

Traditional uses: Native Americans used the root as a ceremonial fetish to keep ghosts away. The decoction made from fresh or dried roots reduced fever and induced sweating. The root is considered a panacea in China and Korea as a tonic and an adaptogen—that is, it helps the user to adapt to stressful conditions. It is said to potentiate normal function of the adrenal gland. Ginseng root is considered a stimulant and an aphrodisiac that enhances the immune response and may improve cerebral circulation and function as well as regulate blood pressure and blood sugar. In traditional Chinese medicine terms, it tonifies primordial energy (increases libido). It is a tonic for the spleen and lungs.

Modern uses: Chinese, Russian, Korean, and European studies suggest that ginseng enhances production of interferon. It is considered an ergogenic aid and may improve endurance. It is reported to regulate plasma glucose. Other research focuses on its anticancer, antiproliferative, and antitumor activity against leukemia and lymphoma. Ginseng's antimicrobial and antifungal activity has been demonstrated. (Cold FX is an over-the-counter treatment for colds that contains ginseng. It has proven effective in clinical trials.) Root preparations lower or raise blood pressure. Ginseng is also used as an immune-system stimulant to help resist infection. Preliminary studies suggest it may increase mental acuity, and it has an estrogen-like effect on women. Studies suggest it may protect against radiation sickness and other physical, chemical, and biological stress, thereby supporting its antistress applications. Considered by many the closest thing to a cure-all in nature.

Asian ginseng (*P. ginseng*) is considered warming and stimulating. Red Korean ginseng (*P. ginseng*) warms more than Asian white. American ginseng (*P.*

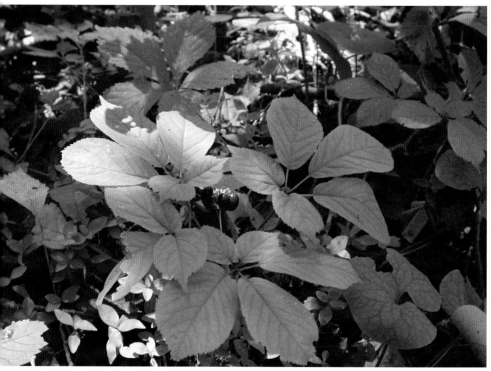

Ginseng, *Panax P. quinquefolius*

quinquefolius) cools, moistens, and soothes. American ginseng is considered a better tonic than Asian ginseng, at least in the eyes of Asian practitioners.

CAUTION: Always use this herb under the supervision of a professional health-care practitioner. Taking more than 3 grams of ginseng per day may cause diarrhea, anxiety, dermatitis, and insomnia. Mild reported side effects include headache and skin rash. Ginseng may strengthen the effects of caffeine. Large doses may cause hypertension, asthma-like symptoms, heart palpitations, and, rarely, dysmenorrhea and other menstrual problems. There have been two reports of interactions with phenelzine, a monoamine oxidase inhibitor. Avoid gin-

seng if you have diabetes, fever, emphysema, hypertension, arrhythmia, upper respiratory infections, asthma, and bronchitis. Chinese practitioners caution against using ginseng with colds (this is in contrast to its proven benefits fighting reinfection with a cold), pneumonia, and other lung infections. Do not use while on internal steroid therapy. Avoid during pregnancy and while nursing until further studies are available.

Notes: Ginseng is becoming rare in the wild. Roots may be ordered at www.herbs.com and from numerous other plant and seed resources. I have found many of my Chinese herbs to harbor eggs and larvae that later emerged as some exotic and startling variety of flying insects and fast-moving beetles. Ginseng roots imported from China are now sprayed with fungicide. Scrub these roots thoroughly before grinding them for use.

Use an old sausage grinder to grind hard, dried roots into powder (the dried root is tough enough to break blades of an electric pepper mill!). My typical dose is 3 grams in decoction. Simmer for thirty minutes. Or put a 60- to 100-gram root (cut to fit) in 1 liter of spirits (vodka, rum) for two weeks. Drink judiciously for its physiological effects. The powdered herb may be purchased; I use 1 teaspoon of powder to 1 cup of hot water twice a day. I drink this for two weeks, then take two weeks off, then two more weeks on. Because I am a hot, type A person, I choose American ginseng (*P. quinquefolius*) for its cooling, calming effect.

Wildlife/veterinary uses: I compound ginseng into three formulas for racing pigeons: pigeon-performance capsules, a nourishing prerace tea, and a cleansing, strengthening postrace tea. The powdered root and root extract is widely used in animal performance formulas.

Goldenseal

Hydrastis canadensis L.

Description: Perennial to 11 inches in height. Bright yellow (golden) rhizome. Two ribbed leaves; lower is typically smaller, sessile; upper leaf on a long petiole, with seven lobes, finely serrated. Solitary flower, found on an erect stem, with three small greenish white petals

that disappear quickly. Fruit scarlet, with one or two black glossy seeds.

Location: Eastern United States. Forest dweller; wet, well-drained soil; in spreading colonies on banks in woods. Often found growing near ginseng. Cultivated nationwide.

Traditional uses: Air-dried rhizomes and root fibers were used to treat diarrhea. Cherokees used root decoction as a cancer treatment and as a tonic and wash for inflammations, infections, and wounds. Goldenseal was also used as an appetite stimulant and to treat dyspepsia. The dried root was chewed to treat whooping cough. A decoction was used for earaches. An aqueous decoction of the root was filtered through animal skin or cloth and applied as eyewash. The root steeped in whiskey was taken as heart

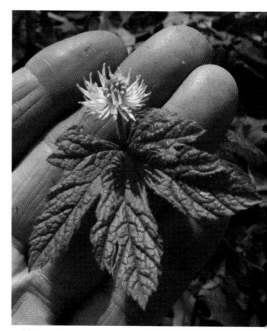

Goldenseal, *Hydrastis canadensis*

tonic. Tuberculosis, scrofula, liver problems, and gall problems were all traditionally treated with the root extraction.

Modern uses: Standardized extracts from air-dried rhizomes and root hairs are taken with water or in capsules to stimulate bile secretion or hydrochloric acid secretion and to hasten and improve peristalsis. The drug has a weak antibiotic and weak antineoplastic (anticancer) activity. It may constrict peripheral blood vessels and is said to stimulate and cleanse the liver. It is used as a therapy for upper respiratory infections. A few holistic practitioners still recommend it as a topical eyewash. Taken internally goldenseal may increase depressed white blood cell counts, as reported in research on traditional Chinese medicine. Clinical trials have suggested its effectiveness against traveler's diarrhea. The root paste is applied externally to treat wounds and fungal infections. Goldenseal's bitter taste may stimulate hunger and be useful in treating anorexia. When using over-the-counter products, seek professional advice and follow directions on the package.

CAUTION: Do not take goldenseal if you are pregnant or lactating due to the uterine-stimulating activity of plant alkaloids and insufficient data on breast milk and alkaloid secretions. Goldenseal is extremely bitter and may be rejected for that reason by some. It is nontoxic at recommended dosages; however, large doses of the physiologically active chemicals in goldenseal—berberine and hydrastine—may be fatal. Amounts in excess of the therapeutic dosages may cause stomach upset, nervousness, and/or depression. Large doses may cause hypertension, involuntary reflex action, respiratory failure, convulsions, paralysis, and death. The herb may negate the activity of heparin, as reported for the isolated alkaloid berberine.

Notes: Goldenseal is scarce in the wild due to overharvesting. Many botanical gardens exhibit goldenseal, and the plant is widely cultivated in the United States and Canada. Personally, I don't see goldenseal as a particularly useful herb. There are safer, more efficacious herbs for the same ailments. I rely more on echinacea, Siberian ginseng, and astragalus. I have used goldenseal for treating athlete's foot by mixing equal amounts of cinnamon, oregano, and goldenseal powder; moistening the mixture with alcohol; and then applying it with a Q-tip to areas of the foot and between the toes. My dentist's dissertation measured the antimicrobial activity of goldenseal root powder in vitro and found the alkaloids weakly antimicrobial.

Wildlife/veterinary uses: Goldenseal is one of several natural products in Brain Cool, an herbal supplement that the manufacturer claims helps rebuild nerves in horses. It is also used in training mixes, wound treatment, and fertility-enhancing formulas for horses. Goldenseal is a vital component in the postrace cleansing formula I compound for racing birds.

Skullcap

Scutellaria baicalensis; S. lateriflora L.

Description: Perennials, eight species. *S. lateriflora* grows to 3 feet in height. Leaves opposite, oval to lance shaped, toothed. Flowers blue violet, lipped and hooded; grow from leaf axil on racemes.

Location: East of the Mississippi; various species across the West. Wet mature woods, thickets. *S. baicalensis,* cultivated as a drug in Oregon and elsewhere, has escaped to the wild.

Food: Not edible; toxic.

Traditional uses: *S. lateriflora* was used by the Cherokees for dysmenorrhea and to promote menstruation. A decoction of plant was taken to dispel afterbirth. A powdered root infusion was used to clean the throat. Historically *S. lateriflora*'s antimicrobial tea was used to treat rabies successfully, and the tea is considered antispasmodic and sedative.

Modern uses: *S. baicalensis* is primarily used for diarrhea and dysentery. It may affect liver function in a positive way due to anti-inflammatory bioflavonoids. *S. barbata* is used as a detoxicant of the liver for various poisonings. *Baicalensis* is used as a febrifuge; it is considered hypotensive and may lower cholesterol levels. It is antispasmodic, a cholagogue (stimulates liver), stems bleeding, and has a mild diuretic effect.

CAUTION: Unspecified doses may be toxic. Use skullcap only under the supervision of a professional holistic health-care provider.

Notes: This is a favorite sedative in the hands of Northwest School of Naturopathic Physicians.

Wildlife/veterinary uses: A Polish study demonstrated that the addition of the ground root of *S. baicalensis* fed to chicken broilers essentially changed the level of calcium and iron in relation to the control group in the blood serum in sixth week of the birds' life (see Króliczewska and Zawadzki, "The Influence of Skullcap Root Addition . . . ," appendix D).

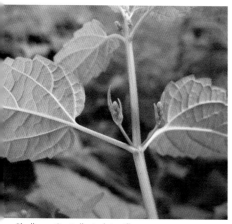

Skullcap, *Scutellaria lateriflora*

Mistletoe, Injerto

Phoradendron tomentosum; also called *P. macrophyllum* (Engelm.) Cockerell

Description: Parasitic epiphyte. Thick branched, semievergreen, growing parasitically on the branches of blue oak, valley oak, and other oak trees. Leaves oblong to ovate to 3 inches. Berry whitish to translucent.

Location: Texas to California. Wooded roadsides, plantation gardens, yards. Parasitic on mesquite, hackberry, ash, oak, willow, sycamore, and cottonwood trees.

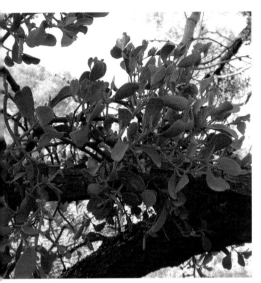

Mistletoe, *Phoradendron* sp.

Food: Not edible; may cause dermatitis.

Traditional uses: Mistletoe is a dangerous abortion-inducing agent (abortifacient) that has killed women. Native Americans considered all parts of the plant toxic, and they are. European pagans used *V. album* (not shown) as a physical aphrodisiac to induce passion.

Modern uses: Most research has been performed on European mistletoe, *V. album,* which shows promise as a potential antidiabetic. The extract is used to treat rheumatism and as adjuvant therapy for cancerous tumor treatment. One person with small-cell lung cancer responded to mistletoe therapy and lived for more than five years (Bradley and Clover, *Thorax* 44 [1989]: 1047).The tea from *V. album* is considered hypotensive and may be effective against asthma, diarrhea, tachycardia, nervousness (as a nervine), amenorrhea, whooping cough, and epilepsy. The whole, cut, and powdered herb is used, but because of its toxic nature, seek consultation with your holistic health-care physician.

CAUTION: All parts are considered toxic. People have died from drinking the berry tea.

Notes: These parasitic epiphytes are easily found on live oaks along two-lane roads heading into Abilene, Texas. *P. tomentosum* raises blood pressure and increases uterine and intestinal motility, whereas *V. album* reduces blood pressure and is calming and antispasmodic. But the chemistry of the two species is virtually identical, which suggests that the activity in vivo may be dose dependent.

Wildlife/veterinary uses: West Texas ranchers have used mistletoe growing on mesquite as a survival food for foraging cattle. Bluebirds, robins, cedar waxwings, and other birds eat the fruit. Deer and elk will eat the plant as emergency forage.

CHAPTER 3

Woody Plants of Eastern Forests, Yards, Meadows, and Roadsides

Our cultural perspectives on Nature and our treatment of the non-human are not merely "wrong" in some contrived moral philosophic sense, but monstrous and unnatural.

—JOHN LIVINGSTON, *ROGUE PRIMATE*

The following medicinal plants are found in forested areas of the United States. Bear in mind that biomes often overlap, and you may discover these plants in areas of transition—from field to forest, for example, or the transition zone from forest to marsh or along wood-lined roadsides.

Grapes, Wine, and Grapeseed Extract

Vitis vinifera L.; *V. labrusca* L.

Description: Hairless, scaly vine may climb to 160 feet. Flowers in tight panicle (cluster), yellowish green. Fruit characteristic of grapes bought in a market, but smaller, seedy.

Location: Nationwide in America; also indigenous to Europe and Asia. American wild varieties are found in forest, along forest edges and marshy areas.

Food: Fruit is healthful off the vine, dried as raisins, and prepared as juice or red wine. Add this fruit to your daily diet. Eat organic cultivars when possible.

Traditional uses: *V. labrusca* (fox grape) fruit was used to treat diarrhea. The leaf

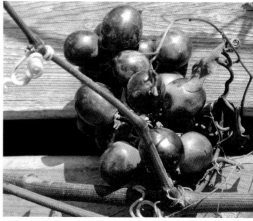

Grapes, *Vitis* sp.

infusion was used as blood-cleansing tonic. Wilted leaves were applied as a poultice over sore breasts. The root decoction was taken to treat rheumatism. An infusion of the shaggy bark was used for urinary problems. A wet poultice treated headaches. Fruit was consumed to reduce nausea and prevent vomiting. Wine of *V. vinifera* may protect the heart.

Modern uses: Grapeseed extract is used as an antioxidant to treat pancreatitis and edema. The extract appears to improve blood flow (venous efficiency) and symptoms related to retinal pathology, including resistance to glare and poor vision in low light (this effect is challenged by recent research). The seed extract may improve microcirculatory function. It is considered a capillary protectant, an anti-inflammatory, and an antioxidant. Grapeseed extract is also used with heart patients to prevent artery damage. This protective feature is due to the protective activity of bioflavonoids. It is used in Europe to treat varicose veins and other compromised capillary blood flow problems due to platelet aggregation, diabetes, and altered blood rheology (blood flow problems). Studies suggest grapeseed extract may induce hair growth. Follow recommended dosages on the package.

The phenolic compounds found in grapes—especially dark-skinned grapes—may improve heart function and mental function and protect against heart disease and Alzheimer's. Ayurvedic medicine advocates eating raisins (dried grapes) for chronic bronchitis, heart disease, gout, fevers, and enlarged spleen or liver. Unsweetened grape juice treats constipation, especially with children. And studies show red wine raises HDL (the so-called good cholesterol) and provides a protective effect, reducing the risk of developing coronary heart disease.

CAUTION: Do not take wine and other alcoholic beverages during pregnancy or while nursing. There are no known contraindications for grapes, grapeseed, or grape juice.

Notes: We grow three varieties of grapes in our garden. To make a tart marmalade, we pick and blend the grapes and then simmer to thicken. Do not add sugar. This produces a freezer jam that is rich in bioflavonoids. Grapes leaves are edible and may be steamed and wrapped around rice dishes, Greek style. Grapes should be eaten raw (grow your own) or lightly cooked or fermented. The unfermented juice may not be as effective as wine for the fruits' antioxidant, capillary protectant, and anti-inflammatory actions. Tannins and other phenolic compounds released from skins provide a more potent mix of protection when formed and released during the fermentation process.

Wildlife/veterinary uses: Grapes and raisins can be toxic to pets when eaten in large amounts (see www.vetinfo.com). Two pounds of grapes caused renal failure in a dog. Grapes are eaten regularly by birds and mammals, such as the scrub jay and eastern fox squirrel.

Oaks
Quercus spp.

Description: The best way to learn to identify oaks is to visit an arboretum. There the oaks will be labeled for identification. Armed with this visual proof, you will be more successful in the bush gathering nuts for the winter.

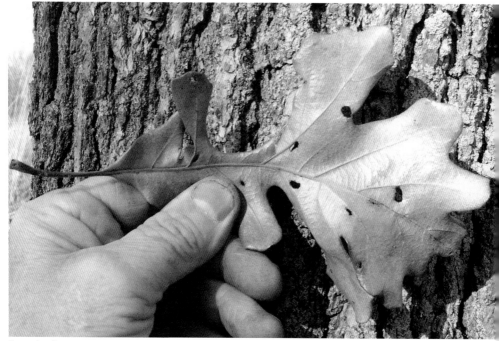

Bur oaks, *Quercus macrocarpa*

Location: Various species nationwide. Yards or woodlots, forested areas, roadsides.

Food: Generally speaking, acorns from oaks that have rounded leaf lobes are less bitter than acorns from species of oaks with pointed leaf lobes. White oak (*Q. alba*), bur oak (*Q. macrocarpa*), swamp chestnut oak (*Q. michauxii*), and chestnut oak (*Q. prinus*) are good examples of sweet acorns from the eastern United States. The chinquapin oak or yellow chestnut oak (*Q. muehlenbergii*) also has bittersweet acorns. Out west look for Gambel's oak (*Q. gambelii*), blue oak (*Q. douglasii*), and Oregon white oak (*Q. garryana*). Black oak (*Q. velutina*) and red oak (*Q. rubra*) are extremely bitter and considered not edible by this author. Tannins in acorn meat embitter the taste, but

tannins are water-soluble phenolic compounds that leach away in water. A quick fix in the kitchen is to puree acorn meat in a blender, using 2 cups of water for every cup of nut meat. Blend thoroughly. Then strain and press the water out of the nut meat through cheesecloth, a clean pair of pantyhose, or a clean white sock. I like acorn mash on baked potatoes, over tomato sauce, in all baking recipes, or out of hand as a snack. Native Americans mashed and sun-dried the acorn meat before using it for food, as drying the meats make them more palatable.

Traditional uses: White oak (*Q. alba*) has tannin-rich bark. Tannins are antiseptic and astringent. Native Americans and pioneers made a tea from the bark for mouth sores, burns, cuts, and scrapes.

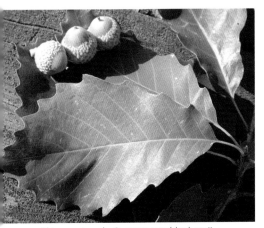

Chinquapin oak, *Quercus muehlenbergii*

The bark extraction, considered a panacea, was believed to provide cancer protection. Dried and powdered bark was sprinkled over the navel of an infant to heal the wound caused by removing the umbilical cord. Red oak (*Q. rubra*) bark in decoction was used to treat diarrhea; the tannins once again account for the reported effectiveness of this remedy. The bark of pin oak (*Q. palustrus*) was prepared in decoction for dysentery and for edema of joints. The inner bark was heated and infused with water by dropping a hot stone into a gourd or skin bag, and the resulting tea was taken for intestinal pain (analgesic). Chinquapin oak (*Q. muehlenbergii*) bark was decocted by people of the Delaware and Ontario Nations to stop nausea and vomiting (antiemetic). Most species of oak bark were boiled and the decoction taken internally for dysentery and diarrhea. And the bark and wood decoction of tannin-rich oaks was used externally to treat inflammations, sores, hemorrhoids, sore muscles, and tender joints.

Modern uses: Oak bark extract, typically from *Q. robur* or *Q. petraea,* is Commission E–approved for treating bronchitis, cough, diarrhea, mouth and throat sores, and inflammations of the skin. Chemicals from oak bark are being tested as a cancer therapy.

Notes: All oak nut meats can be improved by an overnight soaking in fresh water. Native Americans would shell, crack, or smash the acorns then place them in a skin bag and soak them in a stream for a day or two to remove the bitter tannins. Chopping the acorn meats thinly, then drying them, reportedly attenuates the bitter taste.

Wildlife/veterinary uses: Squirrels prefer white, chinquapin, and bur oak acorns but will eat all species. If you want some acorns, better gather them in a hurry. In a "mast" year when oaks produce two to three times their normal acorn crop, we all benefit—especially deer, bear, squirrels, woodpeckers, wild turkeys, and partridges.

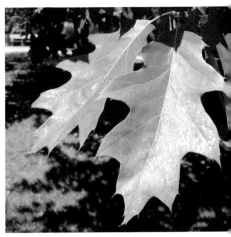

Red oaks, *Quercus rubra*

Maples:
Sugar Maple; Red Maple; Big-leaf Maple, Black Maple

Acer spp.: *A. saccharum; A. rubrum; A. macrophyllum; A. nigrum*

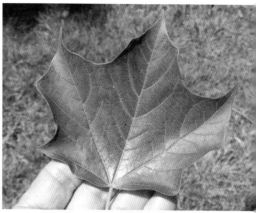

Black maple, *Acer nigrum*

Description: Crowns of trees broad and rounded in the open. Bark smooth when young, furrows with age. Leaves typically three lobed. Red maple leaves have distinctive red petioles. Seeds have the characteristic helicopter-blade appearance and fly accordingly.

Location: Various species broadly diversified throughout the United States and southern Canada. Wet woods, dry woods. Sugar and red maples are generally found east of the Mississippi River; big-leaf maple is a Northwest native. Black maple overlaps the range of the sugar maple in the eastern United States but is somewhat restricted to the upper Midwest.

Food: The winglike seeds may be eaten but are poor tasting. Pluck the seeds from the helicopter-blade husks and cook or stir-fry like peas. You will soon have your fill of them! Maple sugar and maple syrup from the winter and spring sap are what these trees are all about. For taps or information on where to purchase them, contact a maple sugar mill near you (they'll probably sell or give you a few). Using a brace and ⅜-inch bit, drill through the bark until you hit hardwood. Clean the hole thoroughly, then drive the tap in with a hammer. Sap flows best on warm sunny days after a freezing night. In southern Michigan tapping begins in late January and continues until early April,

when the sap runs dark, thick, and stingy. Trees under 10 inches wide require only one tap. For larger maples you may insert two or three taps in a circle around the tree. Use a covered pail to collect the sap. If you're going to boil the sap down on an open fire, make certain your wood is dry, as smoke will give the syrup an undesirable flavor. I use three pans over a long, narrow fire pit, pouring the sugar water from pan to pan as it cooks. Pan number one receives the fresh water from the trees, pan two will receive the reduced water from pan one, and pan three receives the further reduced water from pan two. Pan three, of course, will have the thickest, richest water. Boil the syrup in pan three until it is thick enough to coat a spoon.

Traditional uses: Maple syrup is a glucose-rich sugar substitute with the added benefit of numerous minerals. I prefer it as a sweetener to overrefined white sugar. Traditionally maple syrup has been used to flavor and sweeten cough syrups. The unfinished fresh sap is considered a mineral-rich tonic.

Modern uses: Maple syrup is touted as a good source of minerals, but there are no proven pharmaceutical uses.

Notes: Other trees that may be tapped include black walnut and white, black, and yellow birch. Grapevines climbing high into the forest canopy can also be cut (to save the tree) in the spring to provide copious amounts of mineral-laden water from the wounds. I store a couple gallons of maple water in the freezer and keep one in the refrigerator as a water source that, for flavor and nutrition, beats all those fancy spring, geyser, artesian, mineral, and stuffed-shirt water sources.

Wildlife/veterinary uses: Maple seeds are a favorite spring food for squirrels, mice, and other rodents. Maple water (sap) is a nutrient- and mineral-rich water for domestic and wild animals.

Black Walnut
Juglans nigra L.

Description: Large hardwood tree. Bark ridged, deeply grooved, dark. Large leaves with seven to seventeen leaflets; leaflets toothed, narrow, rough, slightly hairy underneath. Break a hairless twig and note the pith is light brown and chambered. Flower is catkin forming in April or May. Fruit is 1 to 2 inches in diameter, with a round husk over a nut, and nut meat inside that.

Location: Eastern United States. In fertile soil, often lining roadsides where the ample nut crop could be easily harvested.

Food: Nuts are used in baked goods, cereals, waffles, pancakes, and salads. Or eat them on the hoof out of hand. My

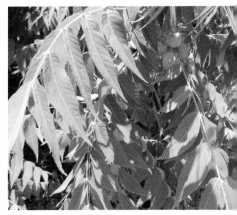
Black walnut, *Juglans nigra*

favorite recipe is black walnut pawpaw fruit chocolate cake (see p. 83).

Traditional uses: Native Americans used the bark, inner bark, leaves, and nut meats. The bark was chewed to treat mouth sores and toothache. Husks of nuts and the crushed leaves were used to treat ringworm. The decoction of bark is emetic. An infusion of nutshells was used as a wash over itchy inflammations. Oil from the nut was used as lotion and hair oil. Charred twigs, sticks, and bark were applied to wounds, burns, bites, and the sap was applied to bites and inflammations (see Moerman, *Native American Ethnobotany;* appendix D).

Modern uses: Black walnut husk extract is antifungal. An antifungal compound can be made by combining equal parts of tincture of goldenseal, cinnamon, tea tree oil, and black walnut husk tincture. Black walnuts as health food are little studied, but research from Loma Linda University on English walnuts (California walnuts) demonstrated a positive cholesterol reducing-ability. Participants ate 20 percent of calories from walnuts, and their ratio of LDL to HDL was lowered by 12 percent (*Nutrition Today* 30, no 4 [1995]: 175–76). Walnuts may help prevent hyperthyroidism and scabies and may lessen the inflammation of psoriasis and arthritis. Walnuts are rich in mood-enhancing serotonin, and they may improve satiety by reducing cravings, thereby treating obesity.

Notes: To remove the husk—the stain-producing covering of the walnut—put the walnuts on a paved driveway and roll them under your shoe. Or jack up a car about 1 inch off the ground, engage the transmission, and shoot the walnuts under the tire. Some people wear gloves and use a hammer to pound and tug the husk away. In my video *Trees, Shrubs, Nuts and Berries* (see appendix D), you can see a simple electric walnut huller in action. A few front-porch, rocking-chair yarn spinners say that walnut husk oil will dye your hair and may even produce new growth. Plants struggle to grow in the toxic soil beneath a walnut tree.

Wildlife/veterinary uses: Nuts are relished by squirrels and field mice. The husks contain a toxic alkaloid and thus have been crushed into dammed streams and used to stun fish. Black walnut extract is used in several natural product wormers for horses.

Cherries:
Black Cherry; Chokecherry
Prunus spp.: *P. serotina* Ehrh.; *P. virginiana* L.

Description: Black cherry trees may exceed 80 feet in height. Bark is rough, scaling: Peel the bark and the wood looks

reddish underneath. Black cherry leaves are ovate to lance shaped, toothed, smooth on top, paler underneath; midrib vein underneath has hairs. Berries are black. Chokecherry is a smaller tree or shrub. Leaves are more oval, sharper toothed than black cherry; no hairs on midrib. Chokecherry flowers are white with a thicker raceme. Berries are reddish. Bark of wild cherry when freshly torn is aromatic, whereas chokecherry is not. Berries of both species hang from long, drooping racemes.

Location: Black cherry: eastern forests from Georgia and Texas north to Canada. Chokecherry: nationwide; often along roadsides.

Food: Black cherry and chokecherry have edible fruit. But the bark, root, and leaves contain toxic glycoside prunasin (hydrocyanic acid) and are inedible. Fruit from both plants makes excellent jams and preserves. Put the whole fruit on cereal, but do not eat the seeds. Fruit may be dried and frozen for later use as a

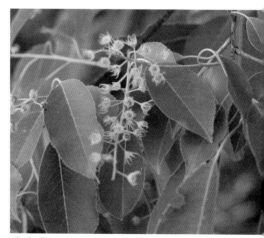

Black cherry, *Prunus serotina*

trail food. Preserves are good for flavoring unsweetened, raw yogurt.

Traditional uses: The inner tree bark and fruit of black cherry were collected in the autumn and used as medicine. First Peoples used a decoction of the black cherry as a sedative and to treat colds, fevers, worms, burns, measles, and thrush. Pioneers took the bark infusion in decoction to treat diarrhea, bronchitis, coughs, and indigestion.

Modern uses: The inner bark of black cherry is used as a flavoring agent and is considered therapeutic for colds, sore throats, diarrhea, respiratory infections, and congestion as well as for external and internal inflammations. These uses are unproven, and little in the way of research has been done on this drug.

CAUTION: Use professionally prepared formulations under the care of a professional holistic physician.

Notes: Black cherry or wild cherry cough drops are still my favorite cough antidote.

Wildlife/veterinary uses: Cherries are important food for birds, raccoons, bears, skunks, and porcupines.

Sassafras
Sassafras albidum (Nutt.) Nees

Description: A small to medium tree. Leaves mitten shaped. Twigs and root aromatic, odor somewhat like root beer. Flowers are yellow green.

Location: Eastern forests and midwestern and prairie states. Located along edges of woods, in drier, well-drained areas as a first growth companion with

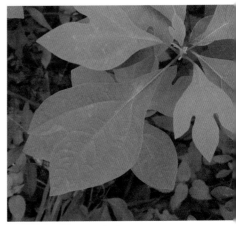
Sassafras, *Sassafras albidum*

oak and hickory in eastern forests.

Food: Spring leaves are dried and used as filé in gumbo and other Cajun dishes. Simply crush the dried leaves to powder and use as a spice. Spread the leaf powder on pasta, soup, cheese, and other savory dishes. For root tea, peel the root, discard the peel, and boil the pith.

Traditional uses: Extracts were used to make perfume and root beer. The root oil was used as an antiseptic until 1960, when the USDA declared it unsafe because of the content of safrole, a carcinogen. The root decoction was used in traditional healing as a drinkable tonic and blood purifier to relieve acne, syphilis, gonorrhea, arthritis, colic, menstrual pain, and upset stomach. Bark tea was used to cause sweating.

Modern uses: Sassafras has no proven effect as a medicine, and because of the toxic effects of safrole, the root tea should be taken judiciously. Small amounts of the dried leaves of spring are still used as a spice.

CAUTION: Sassafras oils may be carcinogenic.

Notes: When camping, I use the twigs as a toothbrush (chew stick). Chew the end of the twig until it is bristly, then "worry" the bristles between teeth and gums. Slippery elm twigs, rich in antioxidants, also make fine chewing sticks. The flavor is refreshing and the sap is a mild sialagogue (promoting the secretion of saliva).

Wildlife/veterinary uses: Turkey, bears, and birds eat the berries; rabbits and deer chew on the twigs—and so do I.

Hawthorn

Crataegus spp.: *C. laevigata* (Poiret) DC.; *C. monogyna* Jacquin Emend.; *C. oxyacantha; C. douglasii* Lindl; *C. macrosperma* Ashe

Description: Shrubs to small trees from 6 to 20 feet in height, many branched. Branches thorny. Yellow green leaves glossy, three to five lobed, with forward-pointing lobes and serrated leaf edges. Numerous white flowers in terminal clusters, with ten to twenty stamens that give rise to small applelike fruit. Fruit ovoid to round, red or black, mealy. There is one seed in each chamber of the ovary.

Location: Hawthorn species are found nationwide. *C. macrosperma:* United States east of the prairie. Damp woods and fringes of forests.

Food: The fruit may be eaten out of hand. It's mealy and seedy, but its heart-protecting value makes it worth the trouble. The fruit may be sliced and dried and decocted or infused in water to make a health-protecting drink. It blends taste-fully with green tea. Berries are gathered in August and immersed in boiling water for thirty seconds and then cut in half, seeds removed, and dried in a food dryer. Berries may be cooked in hot cereals, added to tea. . . . Be creative.

Traditional uses: Hawthorn has long been used to treat heart disease in Europe and China. The active phytochemistry includes bioflavonoids that improve peripheral circulation to the heart and the extremities, including the brain. They also improve coronary blood flow and are hypotensive. Native Americans chewed the leaves and applied the masticated mash to sores and wounds as a poultice. Shoots were used in infusion to treat children's diarrhea. Thorns were thrashed on arthritic joints as a counterirritant. The Okanagan-Colville Nation's herbal art included burning the thorn down to the patient's skin, not totally unlike incense burning (moxibustion) on Chinese acupuncture needles to heighten effect. A decoction of new shoots was used to wash mouth sores. Numerous other remedies are discussed in Moerman's *Native American Ethnobotany* (see appendix D).

Modern uses: Most studies have been on *C. laevigata* leaves, fruit, blossoms, and new end growth. Hawthorn is said to improve and protect cardiac and vascular function by dilating coronary blood vessels and initiating heart muscle regeneration. The extract may be antiangina and improve Buerger's disease (paraesthesia of foot or single toe, an arterial spasm). It's also used to treat tachycardia. Hawthorn is considered cholesterol low-

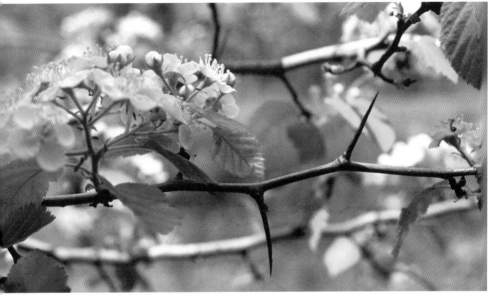

Hawthorn, *Crataegus* sp.

ering and hypotensive. The anthocyanidins and proanthocyanidin fraction are said to be synergistic with vitamin C. In European studies, use of the standardized extract improved exercise tolerance in heart patients. Other studies suggest that the extract may alleviate leg pain caused by partially occluded coronary arteries.

Chinese practitioners decoct the dried fruit and use it for treating irritable bowel and gallbladder problems. The berry is considered antibacterial to shingella (dysentery) species. A decoction of dried fruit is considered antidiarrheal and helpful in treating dyspepsia.

CAUTION: Not recommended during pregnancy and lactation. Proanthocyanidins have been shown not to be mutagenic when tested by means of the Ames test (a standardized measure of carcinogenicity). Safety with berry extracts is well established.

Notes: Some herbs with circulation-stimulating properties in addition to hawthorn include garlic, ginger, ginkgo biloba extract, and cayenne. On my brother's farm grows about a dozen hawthorn trees that have the biggest, sweetest fruit I have ever tasted. In spring we cut off a few dozen clusters of flower buds and emerging new-growth leaves to make a tea. The hot water extracts the bitter bioflavonoids that are hypotensive and antiangina. I have decocted fresh flower tops and experienced flushing and lightheadedness. Perhaps the decoction was too concentrated—I definitely felt enhanced peripheral circulation in the form of face flushing.

Wildlife/veterinary uses: The berries are a valuable wildlife food. Squirrels and game birds relish this fruit. Harvest them first or lose out! Hawthorn also serves as a nesting tree and wildlife habitat. Hawthorn extract has been indicated as a possible therapy for senile pets. Consult your veterinarian.

Pines:
White Pine; Pinyon Pine; Scotch Pine

Pinus spp.: *P. strobus* L.; *P. edulis*; *P. sylvestris* L.

Description: Evergreen trees with medium to long needles. Needles in clumps of five, light green. Pinyon pine is a stubbier plant isolated in dry alpine areas of the four-corner region north to Canada. Its cones harbor the delicious pine nut used to make pesto.

Location: White pine: eastern United States. Pinyon pine: dry plateaus from Mexico north to Canada. Scotch pine: planted as an ornamental in yards, fencerows, and fallow fields.

Food: White pine needles may be made into a tea. I take a handful of needles, crush them, and add them to a gallon jar of water containing mountain mint, lemon thyme, and lemon balm. Squeeze in juice of half a lemon and let the mixture infuse in the refrigerator for six hours. Uplifting! Seeds from pinecones may be eaten. Pinyon pine provides the most notable edible seeds.

Traditional uses: Pine sap is styptic and wound sealing and was used by pioneers and First Peoples to treat gunshot wounds, cuts, scrapes, and lacerations.

There is historical evidence that the presence of antiscorbutic quantities in pine needles helped prevent scurvy, which supports the historical tradition of drinking pine-needle tea.

Modern uses: Oil from the needles of Scotch pine shoots is Commission E–approved to prevent infection and to treat blood pressure problems; colds, coughs, and bronchitis; fevers; oral and pharyngeal inflammations; and neuralgias.

Notes: I brew a tea from all of these pines, mixed with lemon balm, mint, fennel, and lime juice. It's invigorating and anti-infective. This brew is made overnight by cold infusion. Stuff the leaves into a gallon jar, fill the jar with pure water, refrigerate for twelve hours, then drink. Pinyon pine nut ice cream, served in Guanajuato and Dolores Hidalgo, Mexico, is one of my favorite treats. Chop some pine nuts, mash them into vanilla ice cream, and let them infuse overnight. Terrific!

Wildlife/veterinary uses: Squirrels and rodents eat the seeds and make nests

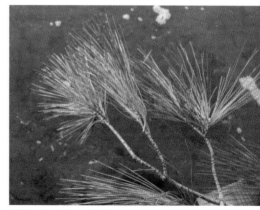

White pine, *Pinus strobus*

with the needles. Doves prefer to nest in pines and spruce.

Poplars: Balsam Poplar; Aspen; Cottonwood
Populus spp.: *P. balsamifera* L.; *P. tremuloides* Michx.; *P. deltoides* Bartr. ex Marsh

Description: Many poplars have ovate leaves on long petioles that provide a quaking effect when the wind blows. Flowers are drooping catkins. Cottonwood (*P. deltoides*) when mature has thick, furrowed bark. Aspen (*P. tremuloides*) is distinctive with its greenish white bark and quaking leaves. Balsam poplar (*P. balsamifera*) has broad heart-shaped leaves, 6 to 10 inches, edged with fine teeth; slightly flattened to rounded leaf stalks. New-growth end buds of balsams are sticky (resinous) and aromatic. The young balsam poplar's bark is gray green and smooth; the mature tree has dark, grooved bark.

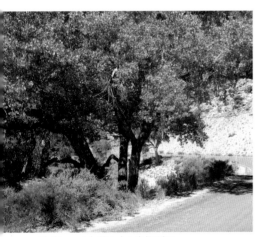

Cottonwood, *Populus deltoides*

Location: Wide distribution in United States. Requires ample water. Balsam poplar is found in the northern tier of states and throughout southern and central Canada. Cottonwoods reside typically in low wet areas. Aspens are found in stands on mountain slopes, in mountain meadows, and along wild rivers.

Food: Balsam poplar cambium (inner bark) is eaten raw. The cambium was boiled, dried, pounded to flour, and mixed with corn flour (masa) and or wheat flour to make bread. Shoots, leaf buds, and catkins taste best when simmered in water. The vitamin C content is high.

Traditional uses: Native Americans considered balsam poplar a panacea: The inner bark decoction was used as a tonic, a treatment for colds and a system cleanser after acute infections. The bark maceration and decoction was used as a wash for rheumatism. Pioneers gathered the reddish resin covering new-growth leaf buds and dissolved and thinned the resin in an alcohol solvent. The resulting salve was applied to seal and heal wounds and relieve inflammations.

Modern uses: Bark, leaves, and leaf buds are used in modern therapies. Leaf bud extract is Commission E–approved to treat hemorrhoids, wounds, and burns. The leaf-bud extract is healing, antibacterial, and antiphlogistic (relieves inflammation). Salicin from the bark and leaves is analgesic (it's considered a precursor of aspirin). The bark and leaves are considered antispasmodic and are used to treat arthritis, rheumatism, and pain and uri-

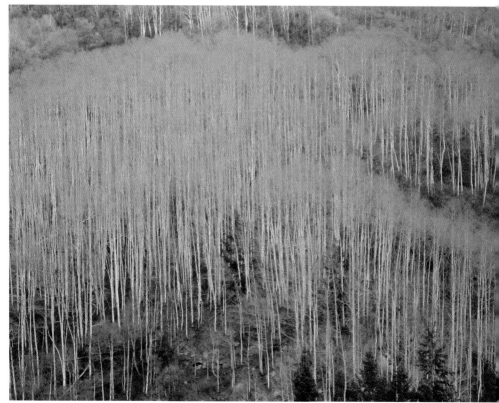

Aspen, *Populus tremuloides*

nary complaints due to prostate hypertrophy. The bitter tonic effect and alterative effect may make it helpful in treating anorexia.

CAUTION: Do not use poplar if you are allergic to aspirin or other salicylates.

Notes: Poplar is not a particularly good firewood. Although poplar tree sap may be tapped, its sugar content is low, and too much boiling is required to sweeten the brew.

Wildlife/veterinary uses: Young trees, leaf buds, and shoots are browsed on by deer, moose, and rodents.

Cedar, Northern White Cedar, Arborvitae
Thuja occidentalis L.

Description: Aromatic evergreen tree to 40 or 50 feet in height. Many branched from the trunk skyward. Flat, scalelike needles to ⅛ inch in length. Cones slender, bell shaped, to ½ inch in length. Heartwood light; bark fibrous with thatched ridges.

Location: Northern states of eastern United States in Canada from Ontario to Newfoundland and Labrador. Swamps, bogs, and coastal areas of Lake Superior.

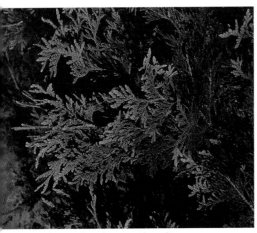

White cedar, *Thuja occidentalis*

Food: Jacque Cartier's French expedition was spared scurvy by drinking the tea from this tree and chewing the needles.

Traditional uses: *T. occidentalis* was named "arborvitae" (meaning "tree of life") by the French when they discovered First Peoples using the bark decoction and leaf tea to treat and prevent scurvy. Eastern tribes like the Algonquin steamed branches to treat colds, fever, pleurisy, rheumatism, and toothache. The fruit was infused into water for treating colic. The Chippewas scarified (pricked with a stick or thorn) charcoal from the burned wood of the plant into the temples to treat headache. Leaf and bark juice was pricked into the skin to treat dizziness and headache. Leaf tea was administered for dysentery and scurvy. The Penobscot Nation poulticed leaves over swollen hands and feet.

Modern uses: *T. occidentalis* is a preferred drug with homeopaths to treat rheumatism, poor digestion, depression, and skin conditions.

CAUTION: Because of its thujone content, this drug must be used with professional consultation and supervision.

Notes: Arborvitae was the first tree to be exported from America to Europe. Soak needle sprays in water and add them to a sauna or steam bath for a relaxing and olfactory experience.

Wildlife/veterinary uses: Red squirrels eat the buds in spring and cut and store seed-laden branches for winter forage. Rabbits, moose, and deer browse on the leaves. Porcupines eat the bark and may inadvertently girdle a tree, killing it. Seeds are eaten by the pine siskin, a small finch of northeastern evergreen forests. Boughs are used as a snake repellent.

Pawpaw, Papaw
Asimina triloba (L.) Dunal

Description: Small, delicate, shade-loving tree. Leaves large, 8 to 12 inches, toothless, lance shaped, broadening toward the tip, terminating in a point; darker green above, lighter underneath. Flowers with six petals precede leaves, and (if pollinated) develop gradually into 3- to 6-inch fruits. Fruit banana to mango shaped, soft and dark brown when ripe. Harvested in Michigan in early October, earlier farther south.

Location: Texas east to Florida and north to Iowa, Illinois, Michigan, and New Jersey. Understory in mature forests.

Food: The fruit is eaten fresh. Unripe fruit will ripen in a few days or a couple of weeks, but when ripe the soft fresh fruit will keep only a couple of days in the refrigerator. The flavor is sweet, intense, and mangolike—loved by many, distained by a few. The fruit may be eaten with ice cream or blended into milk shakes, but it's best eaten fresh from the tree. Or try five pawpaws blended into a Betty Crocker chocolate cake mix. Stud the mix with black walnuts and precooked wild rice. Follow the cake box directions, but cook for an additional three to five minutes. Good Lord, is it delicious!

Traditional uses: Cherokees and Iroquois ate the fruit. The fruit was sometimes smashed and dried into small cakes for winter use. When reconstituted, the dried fruit was blended into corn masa to make corn bread. The inner bark was used to make cordage. Medicinal uses are undocumented.

Modern uses: Research by Jerry McLaughlin at Purdue University may yield a potent anticancer chemical from the leaves and stems of the plant.

Notes: Pawpaw trees are protogynous; that is, the stigma of the flower (the female receptive organ) ripens before the pollen, thus the tree cannot self-pollinate.

Hand pollination is accomplished with difficulty due to the tall, frail nature of the tree. Fruits are located out of reach, and the delicate trees won't hold a ladder safely. In the fall shake and pound the trees to fell the fruit. Pawpaws grow under the sheltering canopy of mature maples and beech trees. They are difficult to cultivate and must be protected from direct sunlight.

Wildlife/veterinary uses: Pollination is "touch and go" from flies and beetles that gather pollen from a different tree. Some seasons the pawpaw trees fail to bear fruit due to an infestation of *Eurytides marcellus*, a beautiful butterfly with larval stage that feeds on the pawpaw leaves, and *Talponia plummerian,* a moth whose larva burrows into the flower, causing it to wilt and die.

Eastern Hemlock
Tsuga canadensis (L.) Carr.

Description: Evergreen tree rounded, less spire shaped, maturing to 70 feet or more in height. Bark and twigs rough. Flat needles less than 1 inch long, green on top, white beneath, silvery looking; attached by means of delicate, slender stalks. Drooping cones are small, exquisitely formed, distinctive. Resin smells of turpentine and tastes just about as good.

Location: East Coast west to Minnesota and Michigan. Rocky ravines; dunes; understory, climax species in beech/maple forest.

Food: Hemlock needle tea is a lumberjack's favorite, best infused in fresh maple sap.

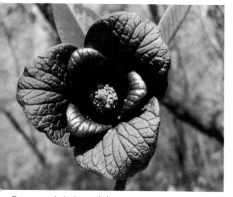
Pawpaw, *Asimina triloba*

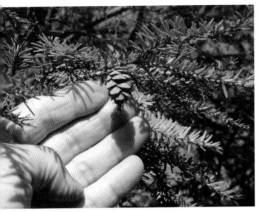

Eastern hemlock, *Tsuga canadensis*

Traditional uses: Native Americans and pioneers used the needles and end-growth twigs in decoction to treat coughs and colds. Wet branches were used over hot rocks in sweat lodges to purge evil spirits and treat arthritis (rheumatism), colds, and coughs. Resin from the bark was used to seal wounds. End branches and twigs were boiled down to form a paste applied externally to sore and arthritic joints. Roots were cleaned and chewed to stem diarrhea. The twig and bark infusion induced sweating. The inner bark was infused and fermented and taken for colds or stomach pain.

Modern uses: Eastern hemlock has no proven modern medical uses, but it is still applied to hot rocks along with cedar boughs in sweat lodge cleansing ceremonies. It is considered a powerful warrior plant (see the DVD *Native American Medicine;* appendix D).

Notes: This sparse and delicate dweller of the Lake Michigan dunes offers a heart-warming splash of green while cross-country skiing through our drab and dunkel winter landscape.

Wildlife/veterinary uses: Squirrels and grouse share the seeds. Needles and twigs are used by rodents as bedding. Deer and hare eat the soft, young buds and new growth.

Balsam Fir
Abies balsamea (L.) Mill

Description: Spire-shaped evergreen to 60 feet in height. At higher altitudes this tree is spreading, low, more matlike. Smooth barked; bark has numerous resin pockets. Flat, stalkless needles to 1¼ inches in length with white stripes beneath, more thickly rounded at the base. Cones purplish to green, to 4 inches in length, scaly, twice as long as broad.

Location: Canada south through the northern tier of the eastern United States. Moist woods.

Food: The needle infusion is a relaxing tea, traditionally considered a laxative.

Traditional uses: Native Americans used the resin to treat burns and wounds and to soothe sores, scrapes, insect bites, stings, and bruises. Tea from needles was

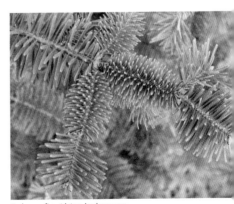

Balsam fir, *Abies balsamea*

used to treat upper respiratory problems: asthma, bronchitis, and colds. Leaves were stuffed into pillows as a general cure-all. Children chewed raw sap to treat colds and sore throats. In sweat lodges, balsam gum was applied to hot, wet stones and the smoke inhaled as a cure for headaches. Branches were steamed to treat arthritis (rheumatism). A bark decoction will induce sweating as a way of treating acute infections.

Modern uses: The resin obtained from bark blisters is considered antiseptic and is an integral ingredient in many salves and lotions, including ointments and creams used to treat hemorrhoids. Proprietary mixtures incorporating balsam resin are sold to treat diarrhea and coughs.

Notes: Balsam wood is used to make canoes, canoe paddles, and cradle boards. For years the balsam has been our favorite aromatic Christmas tree, because its needles are long lasting and fragrant. Balsam gum, a waterproof cement, is used along with pitch to seal leaking birch-bark canoes.

Wildlife/veterinary uses: Deer, moose, and rabbits browse the young shoots and twigs. Seeds are eaten by grouse.

Witch Hazel
Hamamelis virginiana L.

Description: Deciduous small bushy tree or shrub to 10 feet in height, occasionally much taller. Bark thin, brown on the outside, red on the inside. Younger branches haired and yellow brown. Leaves alternate, blunt, indented, with rough margins. Five to seven yellow, short-stemmed

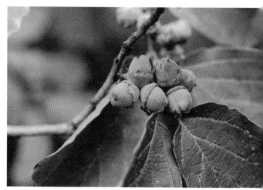
Witch hazel, *Hamamelis virginiana*

flowers appear in clusters before leaves emerge. Flowers grow from the axils of leaf buds. Petals are bright, long, narrow, linear, and roll to a spiral in the bud. Fruit capsule oddly shaped, woody, oval, about ¾ inch long.

Location: Typically east of the Mississippi River. Coastal forests. I have found it growing in Michigan.

Food: Not edible.

Traditional uses: Witch hazel was used by the Cherokee, Chippewa, Iroquois, Mohegan, Menominee, and Potawatomi peoples living in the range of the plant east of the Mississippi. They used the leaf tea externally to treat muscle aches, athlete's foot, wounds, burns, and various skin afflictions. Tea was consumed for coughs, asthma, colds, sore throats, dysentery, and diarrhea. Twigs and inner bark are still used in infusion to treat colds, pain, sores, fevers, sore throat, and tuberculosis. An infusion of twigs was used to treat dysentery and diarrhea. A decoction of new-growth tips and shoots from the base of the plant was used as a blood purifier or spring tonic. Young end tips were used in decoction to treat colds and coughs. Root and twig decoctions were considered a cure-all for just about any ailment: bruises, edema, cholera, and arthritis.

Modern uses: Commission E–approved for external use on hemorrhoids, skin inflammations, varicose veins, wounds, and burns and for mouth and pharynx treatment. Commercial products include liniments, eye ointments, and skin-toning astringents. Witch hazel water is distilled from the leaves and twigs and used as an eyewash and to treat hemorrhoids, colitis, varicose veins, sore muscles, bruises, and sprains. Tannins derived from distilling the active compound are used to treat local skin irritations and inflammations, including eczema. Distilled witch hazel water contains no tannins but is still astringent and is used as a gargle for sore throat and sore gums.

Notes: Witch hazel is commonly grown in nurseries, gardens, and arboretums. Popularly used as a topical astringent, witch hazel is an integral part of an effective wash I blend for psoriasis called Pharmaclean. For more information go to www.herbvideos.com.

Wildlife/veterinary uses: Native Americans decocted the twigs to make an insect-bite wash. They placed a twig in an animal-skin bag, filled it with water, then dropped hot rocks in the bag. The fire-heated rocks provide an instant boil. Water-filled gourds and pottery were heated in the same way. The drug was stirred in, and the wash was applied to bites.

Slippery Elm
Ulmus rubra Muhl.

Description: Deciduous tree to 70 feet in height. Spreading branches with an open crown. Older bark rough and fissured; young branches reddish brown and downy. Leaf buds large and downy. Leaves obovate to oblong, darker green on top, rough to the touch, with a double serrated toothed margin; to 8 inches, typically shorter. Flowers with up to nine sepals and stamens grow in dense, sessile clusters. Spinning top-shaped fruit grows to an inch long.

Location: North America, typically east of the Missouri River. Forests and fields.

Food: The powdered inner bark is dried and made into a beverage to relieve irritated mucous membranes of the throat, stomach, and intestines.

Traditional uses: The inner bark in infusion was traditionally used to treat gastritis and ulcers. The bark extract from this tree acts as an antioxidant and, because it is mucilaginous and demulcent, as an emollient. Externally the extract is an excellent wound dressing, often used on burns and to treat gout, rheumatism, and arthritis. Internal uses included treating gastritis and ulcers of the stomach and duodenum. The outer bark was used to induce abortions.

Modern uses: Slippery elm is still used by holistic medicine practitioners to treat colds, sore throats, and bronchitis. The outer bark is used to make salve. The inner bark is dried and powdered, then added to water and drunk for gastric

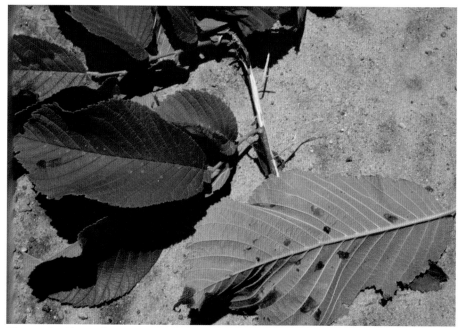

Slippery elm, *Ulmus rubra*

ulcers, duodenal ulcers, and colitis. It is considered antisyphilitic and antiherpetic, claims that are not yet substantially proven. The bark fraction is used in the Essiac cancer remedy, an unproven combination of slippery elm bark, sheep sorrel, burdock root, and turkey rhubarb root. These compounds may be purchased as lozenges, powder, or cut and sifted for making tea as a demulcent for respiratory irritations. See your licensed professional holistic health-care practitioner for consultation.

Notes: Its leaves are rough enough to shave with, but this attractive tree should be added to the garden for its beauty and timeless medicinal qualities.

Wildlife/veterinary uses: Slippery elm is used in training mixes and wormers for horses. One supplemental formula containing slippery elm claims to help maintain joints in horses, and another product for horses called Power Dust reportedly helps heal horses' wounds.

CHAPTER 4

Medicinal Herbs of Wetlands

When I tell you these stories, do you see it, or do you just write it down?

—A ZUNI SPEAKING TO AN ETHNOBOTANIST

These soft-tissue plants are found in wetlands and other low-lying areas, such as marshes, bogs, rivers, lakes, steams, and fens.

Cattail: Broad-leafed Cattail; Narrow-leafed Cattail
Typha latifolia L.; *T. angustifolia* L.

Description: Distinctive perennial to 6 feet tall, lance-shaped wild grass of the marsh. Two hotdoglike flower heads in the spring: upper flower head is male, lower head female. After pollinating, the upper head disperses and disappears. Cattails grow in large stands and colonize handsomely.

Location: Nationwide. Shallow edges of lakes, slow streams, marshes, shallow ponds, any wet and rich ground.

Food: I like to eat the young shoots of spring. New shoots also come up during the summer, and they too are tender after you peel a few layers of leaves away. Sauté the shoots in butter or olive oil. A quick meal can be made by stir-frying the

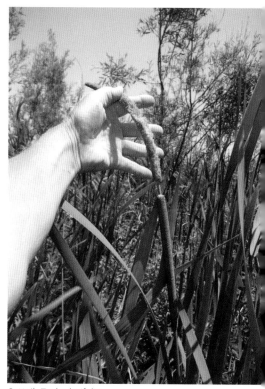

Cattail, *Typha latifolia*

shoots in Italian dressing. The upper (male) flowering head can be stripped in June and used like flour to extend starch dishes: bread, waffles, pancakes, muffins, and corn bread. Male flowering heads are vitamin and mineral rich, complete with essential amino acids. For more recipes see my book *Basic Essentials Edible Wild Plants* (appendix D).

Traditional uses: Cattails roots are polysaccharide rich. Beat the roots into water and use the starchy water as a wash over sunburn. The ashes of burned cattail leaves are styptic and antimicrobial; use them to dress and seal wounds.

Modern uses: Although no longer used medicinally, cattail root provides polysaccharides and, when beaten into clean water, may provide an immune system boost to help prevent acute infections in a wilderness setting. Ash from burned leaves helps seal and keep wounds clean. The dry fluff (cattail seed dispersal hairs) of late-season cattails is an excellent, almost explosive, fire starter.

Notes: Tom, my brother, eats cattail shoots from his property by simply plucking them from the ground and popping them in his mouth. This past spring I tried one. I took a chomp and spit. Some slimy larval insect was residing in the nutritious young shoot. Upon further inspection we discovered that every cattail shoot had a tenant. For years Tom unknowingly had been adding pure insect protein and fat to his high-carb cattail repast! What bug larvae resided there? If you know, shoot me an e-mail at jim@herbvideos.com.

Wildlife/veterinary uses: Dog chow can be made by stripping the old flowering seed heads of cattails and firmly packing them into a quart canning jar. Mix that quart of seed heads in a baking dish with 1 pint of milk, crack in 2 eggs, and combine. Stir in about ½ cup of Parmesan cheese. Bake at 350°F for thirty minutes, then serve to your hound—a well-earned reward after a day of hunting. For more details see my DVD *Herbal Odyssey* (appendix D). Cattail roots and shoots are relished by muskrats, deer, and beaver. Live and dead cattails are used as building material and edible bedding by muskrats and beaver. I have seen porcupines wade into the water to eat cattails and reed shoots.

Reed, Reed Grass
Phragmites communis L.

Description: Tall wetland grass to 9 feet. Root adventitious, growing just under the soil and sending up new shoots as it travels along. Lance-shaped gray green leaves. Flowers borne in the summer on hollow stalk in dense clusters on long panicles, crowned with "hair" that waves in the wind. In late summer the seed head takes on its characteristic plume shape and remains waving in the wind through winter.

Location: Worldwide. Wetlands, lowlands, marshes.

Food: Find the edible shoots in early spring as they pop up around last year's bearded old growth. Peel off the tough outer sheath of leaves and chew on the softer, white-colored tissue, or cook until tender. I like to chew the stalk and suck away the tasty juices. The seeds are edi-

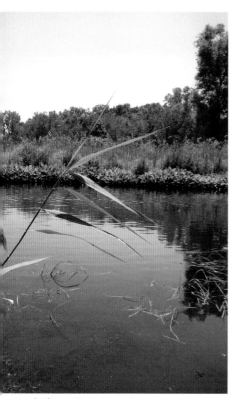

Reed, *Phragmites communis*

ble. Harvest them in late summer and add them to oatmeal, to seven- or twelve-grain cereals, or to other preparations such as bread and muffins.

Traditional uses: The root decoction has mild analgesic effect. In traditional Chinese medicine this herb is prepared in two ways. Method one: The fresh root is simmered in rice wine until the wine is absorbed. The resultant combination is dried, cut, and used in decoction to treat liver and kidney problems and problems related to the heart and kidney meridians, as well as irregular menstruation, insomnia, tinnitus, impaired hearing, diabetes, frequent urination, and allergies. Method two: The root is steamed until

black, cut, dried, and used in decoction for unproven treatments of leukemia, kidney and liver disorders, constipation, diabetes, hepatitis, internal bleeding, arthritis, and rheumatism.

Modern uses: The fresh plant is pounded and its juice collected and applied to bites and stings. The Chinese still practice the traditional uses discussed above.

Notes: The sharp, sturdy shoots can be darn near lethal if you are walking barefoot.

Wildlife/veterinary uses: Albeit not as popular as cattails, reed is a prized food and building material for muskrats, beavers, and porcupines.

Duckweed
Lemna minor L.; *L. gibba;* and others

Description: A hydroponic plant, one of the smallest flowering plants. Forms a green floating cover over stagnant ponds, marshes, and swamps. Its two leaves look like Mickey Mouse ears. Threadlike root hair pulls water and minerals from pond. Sometimes called pond scum.

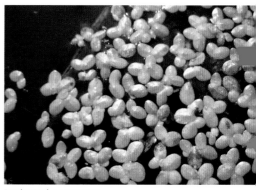

Duckweed, *Lemna* spp.

Location: Nationwide. Ponds, still water, marshes.

Food: The plant can be dried and made into tea. Fresh or dried duckweed may be added to soups or blended into cream soups. Always cook this plant, as its water source may be contaminated. It is virtually tasteless and tough, and small snails and other invertebrates may be enmeshed in the tangle of the plants. Be careful and use sparingly.

Traditional uses: In China the plant is used as a warming agent to treat hypothermia, flatulence, acute kidney infections, inflammation of upper respiratory tract, rheumatism, and jaundice. The whole plant is dried and powdered and then used in infusion or decoction. The Iroquois used star duckweed, *L. trisulca,* as a poultice.

Modern uses: Homeopathically *L. minor* is used to treat colds, fever, and upper respiratory tract infections. Chinese traditional medicine uses the plant to treat acne, epilepsy, edema (swelling), and joint pain in combination with other herbs or with acupuncture as an adjunct therapy.

Notes: When I was working in Japan, I would watch *Lemna* farmers motor over a pond with a long-shafted outboard motorboat that had a screened box around the propeller. The prop was tilted toward the surface, and duckweed was blasted against a screen. When clogged, the screen was pulled and placed in the sun to dry. The hillsides were littered with these screens. The dried duckweed harvest was used as food, animal forage, and medicine. Duckweed produces more pro-

tein per square meter than soybeans and can be used to feed fish, shrimp, poultry, and cattle. Its ability to clean ponds by purifying and concentrating nutrients has made it a candidate for use on sewage ponds. For more about duckweed, go to www.geocities.com/RainForest/Canopy/3631/.

Wildlife/veterinary uses: Hypothetical: *Lemna* tea should be tested for its beneficial effects on cats that are suffering from kidney problems. Duckweed helps cleanse nutrient-rich ponds and provides food for waterfowl and habitat for mollusks, insect larvae, tadpoles, and frogs. It is the kelp of inland ponds.

Mint, Peppermint
Mentha spp.: *M. piperita* L.

Description: Many American members of the mint family. Common characteristics include: square stem, leaves almost always aromatic when crushed, typically aggressive and spreading. Root a spreading rhizome, with square, erect stems. Leaves ovate to roundish, elongated in a few species, typically serrated. Flowers in dense whorls culminating in a terminal spike of blossoms. Flower colors vary by species: white, violet, blue.

Location: Nationwide. *M. piperita* can usually be found around water, shorelines, stream banks, and dunes of the Great Lakes and around mountain passes, blowdowns, avalanche slides, and wet meadows.

Food: Peppermint is used in teas, salads, and cold drinks; with sautéed vegetables; and as an integral part of the subcontinent and Middle Eastern flavor principles. Romans such as Pliny the Elder used mint to flavor wines and sauces. Mint is excellent in Mexican bean soups or in chilled soups of all kinds.

Traditional uses: Aristotle considered peppermint an aphrodisiac, and Alexander the Great thought that eating the mint or drinking the tea caused listless, unaggressive behavior. Peppermint leaves and flowers are infused in water and taken as a uplifting tea. The extracted oil (as well as the tea) is antiseptic, carminative, warming, and relieves muscle spasms. An infusion increases perspiration and stimulates bile secretion. Menthol and menthone, peppermint's inherent volatile oils, are antibacterial, antiseptic, antifungal, cooling, and anesthetic to the skin.

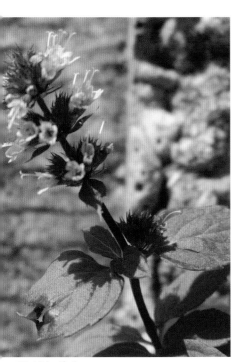

Mint (Mentha)

Modern uses: Leaf and flower extraction are Commission E–approved for treating dyspepsia, gallbladder, and liver problems. Peppermint oil is approved for colds, coughs, bronchitis, fevers, mouth and larynx inflammations, infection prevention, dyspepsia, and gallbladder and liver problems. Recent studies in Europe suggest it may be a treatment for irritable bowel syndrome. The tea and oil have an antispasmodic effect on the digestive system. Peppermint is also used to treat colic, cramps, and flatulence. It may help relieve diarrhea, spastic colon, and constipation. Headache due to digestive weakness may be relieved by taking peppermint, and trials using the extract to treat tension headaches look promising (the essential oil is diluted and rubbed on the temple to relieve headaches and tension). The diluted oil is used in aromatherapy for treating headache and as an inhalant for respiratory infections (i.e., rubbed on the chest as in Vick's Vaporub). Enteric coated capsules are used for irritable bowel syndrome and to relieve colon spasms during enema procedures.

CAUTION: In too high a concentration, the oils are a skin irritant and may burn. Be careful.

Notes: Peppermint, spearmint, mountain mint, and other mints have edible flowers and leaves that may be used in salads and desserts. Try mint blossoms on sliced pears. Mint is a carminative herb used to dispel gas. For a dollar or so buy mint lozenges (Altoids) and use them to alleviate gallbladder pain and pain from a spastic colon. The mint lozenges may quell the discomfort from irritable bowel syndrome. Gardeners beware: Grow mints in a buried steel container to prevent their unabated spread.

Wildlife/veterinary uses: Historically mint was strewn around floors as a vermifuge to rid the home of pests. Veterinarian products include mint flavoring in dog and cat Dental Clens pads. Several gourmet dog cookies are flavored with mint oil extract.

Watercress

Nasturtium officinale L.

Description: Water-loving plant that grows in floating mats. Grooved stem is tough, fibrous when mature. Leaves alternate, ovate; with paired and lobed leaflets. Each leaflet broader toward the base and about ¾ inch wide, but variable in width; with terminal lobe. White flower, ¼ inch wide, with four petals. Blooms in May and sporadically through summer.

Location: Nationwide. Temperate areas; in or near seeps and springs, along the margins of slow-moving, muck-bottomed streams and creeks.

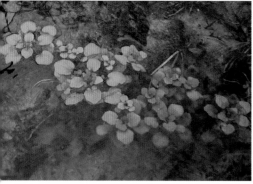

Watercress, *Nasturtium officinale*

Food: Watercress is from the mustard family, and its taste is spicy and pungent. Harvest watercress from a *clean* water source, then cook it. That's right—trust only your backyard if you plan to eat this food raw. You may pull watercress out by its roots and replant it in your garden. Keep it wet and it will reward you with peppery leaves. It is one of the main ingredients in V8 vegetable juice. Watercress is great in Italian dishes: Try it mixed half and half with spinach in spinach lasagna. Sources near me provide edible leaves year-round.

Traditional uses: The pharmaceutical record all the way back to Hippocrates describes watercress as a heart tonic, stimulating expectorant, and digestive. It is good for coughs, colds, and bronchitis and it relieves gas. As a diuretic it releases fluid retention and cleanses the kidneys and bladder. Mexicans revere this plant as a spring tonic. It is dampened and then grilled over charcoal.

Modern uses: Watercress is a good source of vitamins, minerals, and isothiocyanate. The latter may provide protection from cancer and is Commission E–approved to treat coughs and bronchitis.

Notes: Watercress, often found growing wild in questionable water sources, should be relocated to your garden. Keep it well watered and it will cleanse itself. There is a secret place near me, a spring, with more three acres of solid watercress. It is a multimillion-dollar crop living out its life in a hallowed sanctuary.

Wildlife/veterinary uses: Mats of watercress are habitats for snails, insect larvae, and frogs. These creatures attract fish. Should you find a mat on your favorite trout stream, approach cautiously and expect to be surprised.

Horsetail, Scouring Rush, Equisetum

Equisetum hyemale L.; *E. arvense* L.

Description: Perennial to 3 or 5 feet in height. Appears in the spring as a naked segmented stem with a dry-tipped sporangium (spores may be shaken from it). Later the sterile-stage stem arises, with many long needlelike branches arranged in whorls up the stem.

Location: Nationwide. Around marshes, fens, bogs, streams, lakes, streams, rivers.

Food: Native Americans of the Northwest eat the tender young shoots of the plant as a blood purifier (tonic). The tips (strobili) are boiled and eaten in Japan. Mix them with rice wine vinegar, ginger, and soy and enjoy. The roots are eaten by Native Americans in the Southwest.

Traditional uses: Mexican Americans use the dried aerial plant parts of horsetail in infusion or decoction to treat painful urination. Equisetonin and bioflavonoids in the plant may account for its diuretic effect. Native Americans used a poultice of the stem to treat rashes of the armpit and groin. An infusion of the stem was used by the Blackfoot Indians as a diuretic. Cherokees used the aerial part infusion to treat coughs in their horses. An infusion of the plant was used to treat dropsy, backaches, cuts, and sores. Baths of the herb were

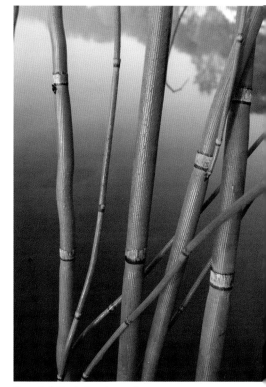

Horsetail, *Equisetum hyemale*

reported to treat syphilis and gonorrhea. This is one of the First Peoples' most widely used herbs.

Modern uses: Commission E–approved externally for wounds and burns and internally for urinary tract infections and kidney and bladder stones. Available over the counter.

CAUTION: An overdose of the herb may be toxic. Use only under the supervision of a skilled holistic health-care professional.

Notes: When we were kids, my brother and I called this plant snakeweed. The segmented stem can be pulled apart and put back together at the joints to make necklaces and bracelets. This fast-

95

spreading garden plant does well in the shade or sun and makes an interesting addition to a flower arrangement. Use the stems to clean pots and pans when camping because it is high in silica.

Wildlife/veterinary uses: Ingestion of horsetail by grazing animals has caused weight loss, weakness, ataxia, fever, and other symptoms. The Meskwaki peoples fed the plant to wild geese and claimed it fattened them within weeks.

Angelica
Angelica atropurpurea L.

Description: Biennial to 9 feet. Stem thick, erect, purple. Large compound leaves divided into three to five leaflets with hollow petioles. Upper leaves sheathed as they emerge, sheath remains around the petioles. Greenish white flowers grow in umbrellalike clusters.

Location: Northern tier of United States, typically east of the Mississippi River. Wet lowlands, along streams and rivers.

Food: Whereas there is little literature on the edibility of *A. atropurpurea,* a similar Chinese herb, *A. sinensis* (dong quai), is eaten as root slices added to stir-fries or soups. A favorite eye-opener and "lip flapper" is a yin and yang cordial. To prepare it, combine 100 grams of *A. sinensis* root (typically available at an Oriental market or drugstore) with 100 grams of whole ginseng root. Add this to ½ liter of peppermint schnapps. Saponins (phytosterols), including phytoestrogens, are drawn from the roots into the schnapps. It takes at least three weeks to get a good tincture. I use the cordial as an aperitif

that balances yin and yang and boosts energy.

Traditional uses: Native Americans used *A. atropurpurea* root decoctions to treat rheumatism, chills and fevers, and flatulence and as a gargle for sore throat. It was often used in sweat-lodge ceremonies for treating arthritis, headaches, frostbite, and hypothermia. The root was smashed and applied externally as a poultice to relieve pain. *A. sinensis* and *A. atropurpurea* are used differently in Oriental and Western traditions, and there are minor chemical differences between the plants too. Unless stated otherwise, assume that the uses described next are for *A. sinensis*, which may be purchased from www.herbs.com as seed or as dried roots from health-food stores and Oriental markets. The root, a warming tonic, is the number-one female herb in traditional Chinese herbal medicine, and it is used to treat menstrual cramps and may improve scanty menstrual flow. As an antispasmodic it is reported helpful in reducing angina. Like other members of the Apiaceae plant family, angelica contains calcium channel blockers, similar to the drugs used to treat angina. According to Chinese practitioners, angelica improves peripheral circulation to distal parts of body.

Modern uses: German holistic health-care professionals prescribe 3 teaspoons of dried *A. sinensis* infused in water to treat heartburn and indigestion. *A. sinensis* is used by European professionals for treating colic. American naturopathic physicians use both species; seek them out for professional advice.

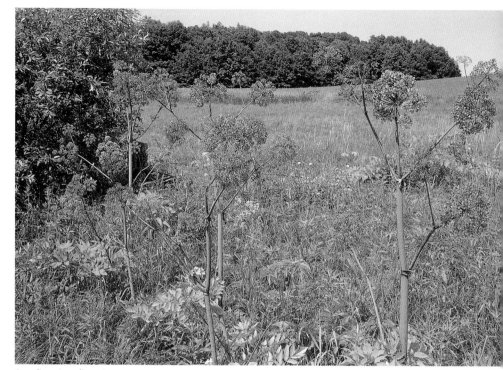

Angelica, *Angelica atropurpurea*

Notes: Angelica roots are used as a flavoring agent for vodka, gin, cooked fish, and various jams.

Wildlife/veterinary uses: Oil from the root attracts fruit flies. Angelica is pollinated by bees, flies, and beetles. The fruit is crushed and decocted as a wash to kill head lice.

Blue Flag, Wild Iris
Iris versicolor L.

Description: Perennial to 3 feet in height. Stems erect, flat, with gray blue tint. Leaves sword shaped. Flower orchid-like (irregular), blue to violet.

Location: Widely distributed east of the Mississippi; also found in the northern tier of western states and southern Canada. Damp marshes, fens, bogs, along streams, edges of lakes. It transplants to the garden and is resplendent.

Food: Not edible.

Traditional uses: The poisonous rhizome was prized by Native Americans as a purgative: It is emetic, cathartic, and diuretic. A decoction of the root was used externally to treat sores and wounds and taken internally to treat colds, cholera, and earache. Algonquins applied smashed roots to burns and used smashed roots as a poultice for wounds. Chippewas poulticed the root over swellings and sores, including scrofulous sores caused by tuberculosis. The root decoction was used for arthritis and kidney disorders.

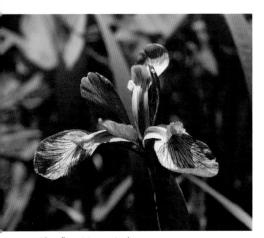

Blue flag, *Iris versicolor*

The Malecite peoples infused iris with bulrush as a gargle for sore throat. Other tribes mixed the smashed root with flour and applied it to painful areas. The Omaha tribe would masticate a root hair, dip it in water, and let the resultant juice drip into the ear to treat earache. According to Moerman (*Native American Ethnobotany;* see appendix D), the plant was viewed as a panacea, good for almost every complaint.

Modern uses: Naturopaths use homeopathic concentrations from the rhizome and root hairs to increase urination and bile production and as a mild laxative. Blue flag is given in homeopathic doses to treat indigestion and skin problems related to liver and gallbladder disease. The herb stimulates these organs, cleanses the body, and is reported to relieve acne, eczema, and other skin disorders related to constipation induced by gallbladder insufficiency. It's also used to treat headaches and respiratory disorders. A few believe it to be a weight loss aid.

CAUTION: Overdose of blue flag may induce vomiting. Never use this plant during pregnancy. The plant juice is a skin and digestive irritant.

Notes: Prior to bloom time wild iris can be confused with edible cattail shoots. Remember that cattail stems do not have the gray to blue tint and are rounded instead of flat. (For details see my book *Basic Essentials Edible Wild Plants* or the CD *Herbal Odyssey* at www.herbvideos .com.)

Wildlife/veterinary uses: Traditionally wild iris has been used in farm animals as a tonic to treat liver problems, jaundice, gallbladder problems, and as a laxative. A standard infusion is made by steeping 1 tablespoon of the dried rootstock in 1 cup of water, then administering the liquid 1 tablespoon at a time twice daily. An alternative preparation was to steep dried root in wine for a half day to produce an extract and then administer it 1 tablespoon twice during the day. Before using the product, consult a holistic veterinarian who is familiar with the plant and can assure you that its toxicity won't hurt your animal (visit http://earthnotes .tripod.com/blueflag.htm).

Jewelweed, Spotted-touch-me-not
Impatiens capensis Meerb.

Description: Fleshy annual to 7 feet in height. Grows in dense colonies. Stems simple, light green, almost translucent, with swollen nodes. Leaves deep green, thin, ovate, with five to fourteen teeth.

Flowers ½ to ¾ inch in length; orange yellow with reddish brown spots; spur shaped, irregular, with the spur curving back, lying parallel to the sac. Fruit is oblong capsule that when ripe bursts open and disperses the seeds.

Location: Widespread east of the Rockies; incidental in the west. Lowlands, wetlands, fens, along edges of lakes, streams, and bogs.

Food: Eat the small flowers of summer in salads and stir-fries. The young shoots of spring quickly form a complete ground cover in wet lowlands and along streams, wetlands, and lakes. Pick the shoots and add them to your mushroom soup and egg dishes, or stir-fry or sauté them with spring vegetables.

Traditional uses: As a traditional treatment for poison ivy, crush and rub the aerial parts of jewelweed over the inflamed area—the plant juices immediately reduced itching as well as inflammation. Jewelweed was used by Native Americans for treating dyspepsia, measles, and hives. The Creek Indians used an infusion of smashed spicebush berries and jewelweed as a bath for congestive heart failure. The crushed flowers were used on bruises, cuts, and burns.

Modern uses: The whole herb infused as an appetite stimulant and diuretic. Naturopaths administer it to treat dyspepsia.

Notes: I grow jewelweed in my garden for greens, edible flowers, and its anti-inflammatory effect on poison ivy, poison sumac, and poison oak. To treat poison ivy, simply crush the aerial parts of the plant and rub them on the rash. Gather jewelweed seeds in fall and spread in a low-lying area of your garden, then get out of the way. It's aggressive and will spread. In the wild it grows in dense colonies often with stinging nettle.

Wildlife/veterinary uses: Jewelweed provides good cover and nesting sites for field sparrows. It may be helpful as a wash for skin inflammations on pets.

Boneset
Eupatorium perfoliatum L.

Description: Perennial to 5 feet in height. Plant rises from hairy, horizontal rootstock. Stems and leaves hairy, rough. Leaves opposite, to 7 inches in length, lance shaped, tapering to a point, fused around the stem at the base. The stem appears to grow through the leaf. White flowers are florets that form large convex head at the top of the plant. Fruit is tufted.

Location: Eastern United States. Thickets and wetlands, open wet prairies, marshes.

Food: Not edible.

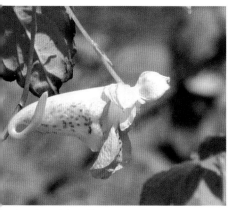

Jewelweed, *Impatiens capensis*

Traditional uses: The leaf tea was considered an excellent nineteenth-century remedy to break fevers associated with acute infections. The leaf tea was considered immune stimulating and used to treat colds, influenza, malaria, arthritis, painful joints, pneumonia, and gout and to induce sweating. Whole aerial parts of plant were applied as a poultice to relieve edema, swellings, and tumors. This Native American cure-all was poulticed over bone breaks to help set bones. Taken internally the infusion of the aerial parts was cathartic and emetic. The infusion was also used as a gargle to treat sore throat. Other uses included treating hemorrhoids, stomach pain, and headache; reducing chills; and alleviating urinary problems. (More uses are discussed in my CD *Herbal Odyssey*.)

Modern uses: Homeopaths use a microdose to treat colds, flu, and other febrile conditions. The dried and commuted aerial parts of the herb when infused in water are reported to be immunostimulating and are taken to fight colds, infections, flu, and other acute infections.

CAUTION: Small doses of the herb are laxative and diuretic, whereas larger doses may induce catharsis and vomiting. Pyrrolizidine alkaloids present in this plant make it potentially dangerous to consume in any form, as these alkaloids have a liver-destroying capacity. Never use boneset without the consultation of a licensed holistic health-care practitioner.

Notes: A striking white flower head makes this plant worth adding to your garden. It provides late-season beauty.

Wildlife/veterinary uses: Grazing animals have displayed toxicity from eating this plant. Symptoms included drooling, nausea, loss of appetite, weakness, thirst, loss of muscular control, paralysis, and death.

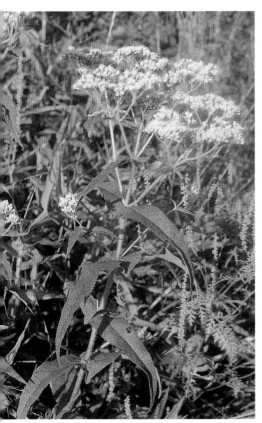

Boneset, *Eupatorium perfoliatum*

Joe-pye Weed; Spotted Joe-pye Weed
Eupatorium purpureum L.;
E. maculatum L.

Description: Perennial. *E. maculatum* grows to 5 feet in height. Long stems purple or purple spotted and leaves hairy and rough; leaves in whorls, three to five,

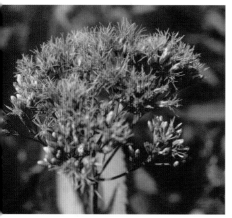

Spotted joe-pye weed, *E. maculatum*

stalked, lance shaped, tapered at tip and base. Large flower head clustered, pink to purple tubular florets. Fruit single-seeded achene. *E. purpureum* is similar: leaf whorls three or four, and fewer flowers in dome-shaped cluster. The roots of *E. purpureum* are preferred as medicine.

Location: Eastern and central United States. Bogs, marshes, fens, wetlands, wet prairies, edges of woods.

Food: Not edible. Some American Indian tribes used the root ash as a spice or as a salt substitute.

Traditional uses: *E. maculatum* decoction or infusion of leaves and root powder was taken internally to treat urinary tract stones and other kidney and urinary tract problems. The root decoction was used to treat bed-wetting in children and as a diuretic to treat congestive heart failure (dropsy). The tea was also used for treating asthma. Native Americans used *E. maculatum* for treating menstrual disorders and dysmenorhea and as a recovery tea for women after pregnancy. *E. purpureum* was used by Cherokees to treat

rheumatism and arthritis and as a diuretic. An infusion of the root is said to be a laxative. Potawatomis used fresh leaves as a wound poultice. Navajos used the root as antidote to poisoning. New England colonists claimed the plant to be a successful treatment for typhus.

Modern uses: Hot infusions of the aerial parts are used by naturopaths to treat colds, fever, and arthritis. The plant is said to be antimicrobial and to induce sweating, loosen phlegm, and induce coughing to remove mucus. It is also used as a tonic and laxative to rid the body of worms.

Notes: Cherokees and other tribes used the hollow stems like straws. The root of *E. purpureum* was used by the Meskwakis as an aphrodisiac (they sucked on the root while wooing). This plant is a striking late-summer bloomer worth adding to your wildflower garden.

Wildlife/veterinary uses: Joe-pye attracts butterflies and is easily transplanted to the garden. For a discussion of how joe-pye weed and other herbs are used to keep pet birds healthy, go to www.holisticbird.org/heal/cs15.htm.

Bittersweet Nightshade, Climbing Nightshade
Solanum dulcamara L.

Description: Climbing vine. Short petioled leaves are dark green, lobed, alternate. Flowers in summer. Purple rocket-shaped flowers. Fruit ¼ to ½ inch, reddish orange, appears in fall. Member of the potato and tomato family.

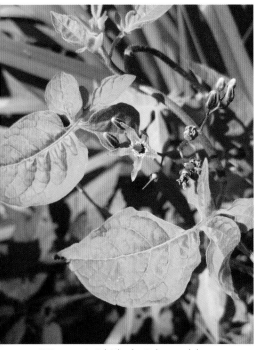

Bittersweet nightshade, *Solanum dulcamera*

and coughing. Seek professional consultation and oversight when considering this herb. Research suggests the herb has anticancer chemistry.

CAUTION: Nightshade is considered toxic, although it is rarely fatal. I have never tried the herb and therefore cannot recommend it. Definitely do not take during pregnancy and while nursing.

Notes: The herb can be gathered in the fall of the year. It makes an attractive seasonal decoration, albeit one that should be kept away from young children who may be attracted to the berries.

Wildlife/veterinary uses: Wildlife and domestic animals may be adversely effected by the toxins in the plant. It's a preferred habitat area for cardinals.

Location: Nationwide. Along streams, ditches, thickets, lakeshores, and bogs. Often clings to willow and other shrubs.

Food: Not edible. Berries are toxic and must be avoided.

Traditional uses: The roots were infused by Native Americans to treat nausea and were mixed with an unspecified herb to treat gas and taken as an antiemetic. Its external use documented in the form of an oil-based salve. It has long been considered an anticancer drug, but this is not proven.

Modern uses: Commission E–approved for treating warts, acne, eczema, and furuncles. Holistic practitioners have used the herb infusion for arthritis, gout, and respiratory problems, including bronchitis

Sweet Flag, Calamus
Acorus calamus L.

Description: Perennial about 2 feet tall. Grows from a rhizome. Stem composed of long swordlike leaves arranged in two rows. Flowers green, on a clublike spadix. Entire plant has intense sweet aroma. Grows in large colonies.

Location: Typically east of the Mississippi. Wetlands, along creeks, marshes, lakes, streams.

Food: Not edible.

Traditional uses: Sweet flag is considered the number-one herb both for medicine and ritual use among seven eastern Native American tribes. The root is a sialagogue; that is, it induces mouth glands to secrete juices. During the Sun Dance ceremony, when First Peoples may sing for ten hours or more, they put a piece of calamus root between cheek and gum to keep their throats moist. Sweet flag leaf garlands were used by Native Americans as fragrant necklaces to mask body odors. The root tea is an appetite stimulant. The aromatic, bitter root was considered a stomach tonic to treat dyspepsia and gastritis. The root was chewed for toothache. Considered for centuries to be a fine nervine, sedative, and relaxant, the root was traditionally chewed or used in decoction by pioneers to treat colds, coughs, fevers, children's colic, and congestion. The dried and powdered rhizome was inhaled to treat congestion. It was considered an antispasmodic, anticonvulsant, and possible central nervous system depressant.

Modern uses: The extract from the peeled and dried rhizome is considered a carminative, tonic, antispasmodic, and stimulant. It increases sweating. In vitro studies suggest that it is anticlotting and that it may aid in treating aggressive and impulsive behavior. The extract is considered antispasmodic and sedative. In Chinese traditional medicine the root extract is used internally to treat gastrointestinal complaints and externally to treat fungal infections. The Asian variety is still considered an aphrodisiac. Triploid strains in

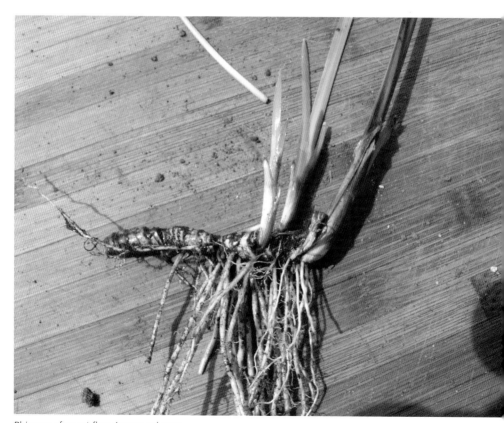

Rhizome of sweet flag, *Acorus calamus*

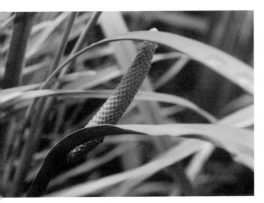

Sweet flag spadix

Europe and the United States are sometimes used to treat ulcers. The triploid strain produces about one-third the amount of beta asarone as the tetraploid strain from India known as kalmus root oil. (Beta asarone is considered carcinogenic.) *A. calamus* var. *americanus* is still used as a bitters to relieve stomach spasms and a distended stomach with concurrent headache associated with poor digestion. According to Chevallier (*Encyclopedia of Medicinal Plants*), *A. calamus* var. *americanus* does not contain asarone. Animal studies suggest that the root extract may lower serum cholesterol.

CAUTION: Beta asarone is a component of *A. calamus* that when taken in ample amounts over time is carcinogenic to laboratory animals. Therapeutic doses of the triploid strain should be monitored. Avoid long-term use. Use only under the administration of skilled holistic health-care practitioner. Follow recommended dosages on the package.

Notes: A few herbalists chew or suck the dried root to keep them awake on long drives. I like to put about a pound of the fresh, crushed and chopped root in a pair

of pantyhose and submerge it in a hot bath or Jacuzzi—it's aromatic and relaxing. If you don't want to kill the plant, crush only leaves and put them in the pantyhose and submerge. In foreign countries the dried and ground rhizome and root hairs are used as a spice and fragrance in food, but because of the beta asarone content, this use is not allowed in the United States. The plant is an interesting addition to the garden, an exotic aromatic used in flower arranging. A particular striking stand is found along the north side of U.S. Highway 12 just east of White Pigeon, Michigan. It has been used by the Potowatomi Nation for hundreds of years.

Wildlife/veterinary uses: The root fragrance may repel some insects, lice, and rodents, but has no effect on the movement of rogue cats and dogs through my yard!

Gentian, Stiff Gentian; Fringed Gentian
Gentiana andrewsii Griseb.; *G. crinita*

Description: *G. andrewsii* is a perennial to 30 inches in height; generally shorter. Stem has four ridges, with clasping oval leaves that embrace the clusters of blue flowers. *G. crinita* has conspicuous fringe atop the petals and is slightly smaller.

Location: Both plants are eastern species found in wet woods, moist fields around wetlands, wet edges of older growth forests, seeps.

Food: Not edible. One European species is said to be an ingredient of Angostura bitters.

Traditional uses: Tea and tincture, a traditional bitters, were used as a tonic, a cooling herb that stimulates digestion and strengthens appetite by means of its bitter taste. Gentian is said to ease stomach pain. The Potawatomis used the herb to treat snakebite. The water made by boiling the root was applied externally to treat backache. Several sources report that pioneers ate the root to stimulate appetite and drank a tea from the aerial parts to aid digestion.

Modern uses: In Europe the entire plant of *G. kochian* is used as a digestive and bitters. Both the European and American species are a liver stimulant and stimulating to the entire digestive system: increasing peristalsis and digestive secretions and promoting improved digestion, assimilation, and elimination. The extract, a constituent in digestives, may be purchased at health-food stores here and in Europe; ask for a stomach bitters with gentian.

Notes: I once saved a stand of fringed gentian that was about to be plowed under to make way for a housing development. These striking plants are most conspicuous in the fall of the year.

Wildlife/veterinary uses: For information on veterinarian use to treat lack of appetite, sluggish digestion, indigestion, and flatulence and to stimulate the liver, see www.denes.com.

Lobelia
Lobelia siphilitica L.

Description: Perennial 3 to 4 feet in height. Oval leaves. Flower distinctive, birdlike, typically blue to blue lavender, throat of corolla white striped.

Location: Numerous species from coast to coast, including subalpine varieties. *L. siphilitica* is found in moist areas, streamside, bogs, fens, wetlands of all sorts.

Food: Not used as food; toxic.

Traditional uses: Lobelia was used to induce vomiting and increase respiration and as a narcotic and analgesic (to treat toothache). *L. siphilitica* was used with *Podophyllum peltatum* (mayapple) to treat venereal diseases. Various species of lobelia were used for treating dysentery, cirrhosis, gastroenteritis, edema, eczema, and schistomiasis. A poultice of root was rubbed on sore neck muscles and back muscles. Both roots and leaves were used as an external detoxifier and analgesic on bites and stings, boils, and sores. A cold infusion of the plant was considered a strong emetic. Lobelia is considered a cure for cigarette smoking, but fatalities may have occurred where the practitioner was not skilled in the use of the herb.

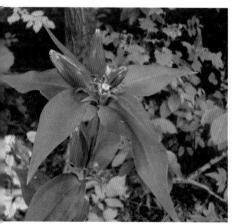

Gentian, *Gentiana andrewsii*

105

Modern uses: Alkaloids derived from various lobelia species have been patented. These include lobeline, lobelanidine, lobelanine, and their various salts. These patented chemicals are potential drugs in treating psychostimulant abuse and eating disorders. The drugs might be used to treat abuse of cocaine, amphetamines, caffeine, opiates, barbiturates, benzodiazepines, cannabinoids, hallucinogens, alcohol, and phencyclidine.

CAUTION: This is a very potent and potentially toxic herb. Do not experiment with it.

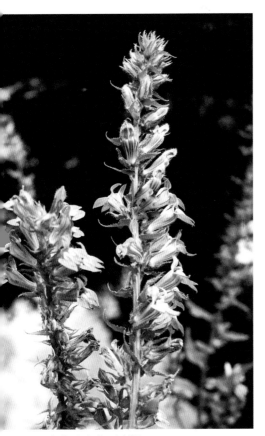

Lobelia, *Lobelia siphilitica*

Notes: Lobelia varieties are found from coast to coast. In western mountains the high-altitude species are much smaller in size and abundant near and above the tree line in the Sierras and the Coastal Ranges. *L. syphilitica* may be transplanted to a moist, semishaded area of your garden.

Wildlife/veterinary uses: A wound treatment formula called Power Dust contains lobelia extract and is used to treat wounds in horses.

Sweetgrass, Holy Grass, Vanilla Grass
Hierochloe odorata L.

Description: Grass 18 to 20 inches tall. Shiny green with solitary stems, purplish base attached to a long adventitious rhizome. Flower inconspicuous, golden yellow, tulip shaped. Crush a leaf and note the distinctive sweet fragrance.

Location: Primarily in the East. Moist meadows, stream banks, bog edges. Prefers sunny locations. Cultivated by Native Americans for ritual use.

Food: Sweetgrass is used in Europe to flavor liqueurs and vodkas. The grain is probably edible but little information about it is available. The plant contains coumarin, an antiplatelet-aggregating compound that may cause excessive bleeding. Sweetgrass oil (coumarin free) is used as a flavoring for candy, soft drinks, alcoholic drinks, and even tea and perfume. Tobacco chews are flavored with the grass, and Native Americans mix

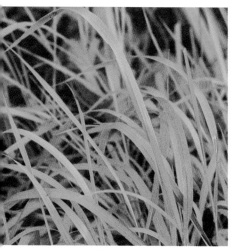

Sweetgrass, *Hierochloe odorata*

the grass with tobacco. Leaf tea is used to treat coughs and sore throat.

Traditional uses: Many Indian nations use sweetgrass for spiritual healing. They burn the grass and dispense smoke (a process known as smudging) and sweep (brush) with the grass. An infusion is used internally to treat sore throats and coughs and externally as wash for vaginal disorders, chafing, or venereal diseases. In Europe it was used in perfumes and sachets and strewn on church steps on saints' days.

Modern uses: Sweetgrass is still used by many Indian nations as a cleansing and purifying agent in sweat-lodge cere-monies. Some Native Americans weave the grass into baskets.

CAUTION: Internal use of sweetgrass should be avoided due to the presence of blood-thinning coumarins.

Notes: Sweetgrass must be contained in the garden because it is invasive. A Native American friend of mine gave me a start of this sweetly fragrant grass. I

placed it in a metal tub to contain its explosive growth. Sweetgrass is great when used in a hot tub, sauna, or sweat lodge. Put a bundle of fresh or dried grass in a sock or pair of pantyhose and immerse the bundle in the tub.

Wildlife/veterinary uses: Flathead First Peoples of the Northwest use sweetgrass as an insect repellent. It can be grown around an odorous pigsty to combat the stench. Although sweetgrass contains coumarins, it is safely made into hay for grazing animals.

Cranberry
Vaccinium oxycoccus L.

Description: Dwarf evergreen shrub 5 to 15 inches in height. Low lying, creeps through bogs on slender stems. Bark hairy to smooth, brown to black in color. Flowers pink; solitary or in couplets, rarely three; nodding, with petals sharply bent backwards like shooting stars. Fruit color ranges from pink to red, depending on ripeness. Small berries are juicy and very tart.

Location: Nationwide in the upper tier of states. Along the floor of sphagnum bogs, in hummocks and wet alpine mead-ows to elevations of 6,000 to 7,000 feet.

Food: You've tried cranberries with turkey. Now try them in your favorite apple crisp recipe—add black walnuts and invite me over. Cranberries also spark up persimmon pudding.

Traditional uses: The berries and berry juice were used as therapy for urinary tract infections—they were reported to acidify urine. Some claim that cranberry

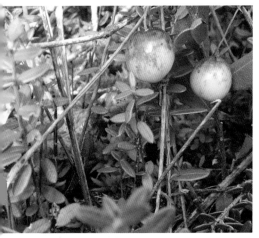

Cranberry, *Vaccinium oxycoccus*

helps remove kidney stones. The juice was also used to treat bladder infections and to prevent recurrence of urinary stones. It contains vitamin C and prevents scurvy.

Modern uses: A study showed drinking the juice may prevent adhesion of *Escherichia coli* to the linings of the gut, bladder, and urinary tract, thus preventing the bacterium from multiplying and inducing disease. In another study 16 ounces of cranberry juice was shown to be 73 percent effective against urinary tract infections. Cranberry juice also functions as a urine acidifier. Cranberries and cranberry juice are used to decrease the odor and degradation of urine in incontinent patients. In one small study 305 grams of cooked cranberries proved effective in decreasing pH from 6.4 to 5.3. In other tests juice showed little effect on pH. However, there is evidence that using the concentrated (no sugar added) juice with antibiotics may help suppress urinary tract infections. I have taken 1 ounce of the 100 percent extract in 6 ounces of water and effectively relieved a urinary tract infection. Of course, this may or may not work for you. The required amount of cranberries or cranberry extract to treat bladder infections and stones has not been established. Seek consultation from your holistic health-care professional.

Notes: There are a couple cranberry bogs in my neighborhood. In October the berries ripen. I dry them in a food dryer or cook them fresh. They are tart and have many benefits. A popular over-the-counter cranberry cocktail juice contains too much sugar. It is prudent to take cranberry extract in pill form or buy pure 100 percent cranberry juice concentrate and sweeten it very little.

Wildlife/veterinary uses: Cranberry is a preferred food of ruffed grouse and cedar waxwing and twenty other species of birds. Fruits hang on the stems throughout the winter and serve as emergency food when other sources are not available. Dead cranberry brush provides valuable cover and nesting sites for birds. NaturVet is a veterinarian-formulated cranberry product providing nutritional support that helps to control maladies of your pet's urogenital system. Cranberry helps to minimize bacterial colonization of the bladder mucosa.

CHAPTER 5

Woody Wetland Plants

Look at a child gently holding an unfledged young robin that has fallen from its nest. Look in that child's eyes. The sweet bondage of wilderness is recoverable.

—JOHN LIVINGSTON, *ROGUE PRIMATE*

This chapter looks at trees, shrubs, and vines of lowland areas, wetlands, lakes, and streams.

Willows: White Willow; Black Willow

Salix spp.: *S. alba* L.; *S. nigra* Marsh

Description: Tree or shrub with lancelike fine-toothed leaves; yellow male flowers and green female flowers in the form of densely blossomed catkins. *S. alba,* sometimes called weeping willow, has drooping branches. *S. nigra* (black willow) is erect, large with shedding branches. Both prefer wet ground and are considered dirty trees in that they constantly shed branches, flowers, and leaves.

Location: Nationwide. Marshy areas, thickets, lakeshores, along streams and rivers.

Food: A tea can be made from the twig bark that contains salicin (an aspirin-like compound). Use the tea with extreme care as salicin and other chemicals released by the infusion may damage your health (see the caution on the next page).

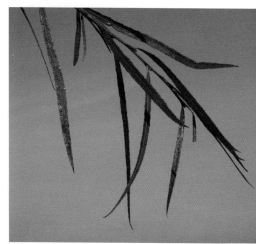

Willow, *Salix* sp.

Traditional uses: Native Americans used the bark of twigs and new growth in decoction to treat tendonitis, arthritis, headaches, and bursitis. An infusion of the stem and leaves releases salicin, the natural chemical model for synthetic aspirin. Aspirin may help prevent acute infections, cancer, strokes, and heart attacks. It may help boost immunity, but it does have numerous side effects and may aggravate ulcers and cause intestinal bleeding.

Modern uses: The extraction, although infrequently used from the tree, is Commission E–approved for treating pain and rheumatism. Not to be used by people allergic to salicyclates.

CAUTION: Much double-blind, placebo-controlled, double-crossover research has been done on aspirin but not on salicin from willow extraction. Keep in mind that the infusion or decoction of willow contains much more than salicin. Recent evidence shows that willow can concentrate cadmium, a toxic metal, in its tissue. All species of willow are known to concentrate this metal when it is available in the soil. I prefer using aspirin for its therapeutic effects.

Notes: Do not garden under or too near a willow. Willow rootlets travel near the surface and suck water and nutrients from the soil. This can distress nearby garden plants. When a willow dies, be aware that the widespread root system has drained the soil of nutrients. Rebuild the soil before you replant the area.

Wildlife/veterinary uses: Cadmium accumulation in the kidney and liver of birds may come from eating willow flow-

ers and seeds. This is especially true of ptarmigan in the mountains near Durango, Colorado; see *Science News* 158 (August 5, 2000). White willow is used in several herbal formulas for horses, a fertility supplement, a joint support complex, and a hoof and foot relief compound.

Blueberry, Bilberry
Vaccinium spp.

Description: Deciduous shrub to 20 inches in height. Sharp-edged green branches. Leaves alternate, ovate and oblong, finely serrated. Flowers greenish tinged with pink, ¼ inch long, containing eight to ten stamens shorter than the styles. Globular fruit blue black, often frosted, with numerous seeds dispersed through the purple pulp. There are numerous species that vary significantly. The terms "blueberry" and "bilberry" may be used interchangeably.

Location: Northern tier states from coast to coast. Wetlands, lowlands, and high-

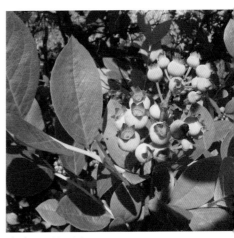

Blueberry, *Vaccinium* sp.

lands, including eastern and western mountains.

Food: This highly nutritious fruit may be eaten fresh or dried. Leaves can be made into tea.

Traditional uses: Native Americans used a decoction of fresh or dried berries to treat diarrhea. The Iroquois used a whole aerial part decoction as a topical application to dermatitis. Bog blueberry (*V. uliginosum*) leaves were infused in water and sugar and taken as a tonic by women after childbirth. Blueberries are a good source of vitamin C and a folk use to prevent scurvy. Dried pulverized leaves were infused and taken for nausea. Other Native American uses may be found in Moerman's *Native American Ethnobotany* (see appendix D). Pioneers used the leaves in decoction for treating diabetes. Berry tea was taken to treat mouth sores and inflammations.

Modern uses: The use of fresh and dried fruits and dried leaves is Commission E–approved for treating diarrhea and inflammation of the pharynx and mouth. The fruit is considered an antioxidant and a capillary protectant that may improve blood flow to the feet, brain, hands, eyes, and other distal areas. It is antiatherosclerotic, antiplatelet aggregating, antiglaucoma, and may provide protection from night blindness. Research suggests it may prevent varicose veins. Blueberry has induced the release of dopamine. And it may be helpful as adjunct nutritional support for Alzheimer's disease.

Notes: Eat a fistful of blueberries daily when experiencing extended periods of bowel discomfort, gas, or diarrhea. Dry the berries in a food dryer and store them in the freezer to treat winter stomach problems.

Wildlife/veterinary uses: Blueberry bushes provide important habitat and food for songbirds, raccoons, and bears. Don't spray them with pesticides.

Elderberry
Sambucus racemosa L.; *S. cerulea* Raf.; *S. nigra* L.; *S. canadensis* L.

Description: Clump-forming shrubs. All four species have pinnately compound leaves that are opposite. *S. racemosa* has five or seven leaflets per leaf, green and nearly hairless above and lighter colored and hairy below. *S. cerulea* leaves are shiny, evergreen in the southern range; ovate or lance shaped with long pointed tips, shorter points and unequal size at base; sawtoothed edges; yellow green color on top, paler and hairy underneath. *S. racemosa* has a red fruit maturing in the summer, whereas *S. cerulea* fruit is blue, also ripening in the summer. *S. nigra* (an introduced European variety and the most studied) and our native eastern variety (*S. canadensis*) are similar. *S. nigra* and *S. canadensis* grow to 25 feet in height. Bark light brown to gray, fissured and flaky. Branches green with gray lenticels, easily broken. Leaves compound, leaflets oblong, ovate, serrated; matte green above, light blue green underneath. White flowers in large rounded clusters. Fruit oval, black to deep violet.

Location: Nationwide. Typically in wet areas, along streams in lowlands and

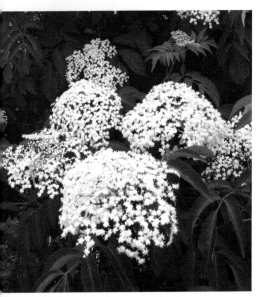

Elderberry, *Sambucus canadensis*

mountains of the West. *S. canadensis* is typically found in wet thickets, along edges of streams, rivers, and lakes in the eastern states and southeastern Canada. *S. nigra* can be purchased in nurseries and transplanted to your property.

Food: Use elder flowers and berries sparingly as food because their safety is not universally established—imbibe at your own risk. We dip the white cluster of blossoms in tempura batter and then cook them like fritters. Sprinkle with powdered sugar and serve as a health-protecting, heart-stimulating dessert. Or cook elderberries, then strain the juice through a sieve, thicken with pectin, and combine with other berry jams and marmalades. The cooked juice may also be added to maple syrup. The juice mixed with brown sugar, ginger, mustard, and soy makes a good wonton dip.

Traditional uses: Flower infusions are reported to lower fever. A wash of the

flowers may reduce fever and be soothing to irritations; it is considered alterative, anti-inflammatory, and diuretic. Flowers and fruit are made into tea for influenza, flu, colds, arthritis, asthma, bronchitis, improved heart function, fevers, hay fever, allergies, and sinusitis. Native Americans scraped the bark and used the root in infusion as an emetic and a laxative. The berry infusion was used to treat rheumatism. The flower infusion was given to colicky babies. Roots were pounded, decocted, and applied to swollen breasts. Leaves in infusion were used as a wash for sores.

Modern uses: Standardized extractions are Commission E–approved for treating cough, bronchitis, fevers, and colds. The therapeutic dose of flowers is reported to be 1 to 3 teaspoons of dried elder flowers to 1 cup of water off the boil. Over-the-counter elderberry extracts indicate the recommended dosage on the bottle. Flower and berry extractions are used to treat acute infections like colds and flu. Herbalist Michael Moore claims that a tincture of the flowers is alterative and diaphoretic, stimulating the body's defense systems. Elderberry flower tinctures may be more effective and more tasteful when combined with mints. The berries can act like a mild laxative, yet at the same time they are antidiarrheal and astringent.

CAUTION: The leaves, bark, root, and unripe berries of *Sambucus* species may cause cyanide poisoning. Cook the berries before consuming them. The western variety, *S. racemosa,* with red berries may be more toxic than the blue and black berries of the varieties *S.*

cerulea, S. canadensis, and *S. nigra.* Avoid eating red elderberries—the fresh berry juice has caused illness.

Notes: Elderberry (*S. canadensis*) grows close to my home; I hop in my boat and can fill two grocery bags with flowers in twenty minutes. Elderberry (fruit) may be dried in a food dryer, then frozen and used in cooking throughout the cold months for disease prevention. I eat the dried berries of *S. canadensis* throughout the winter on cereal, pancakes, waffles, and porridge and in stir-fries. Berries are best when cooked after drying. Flowers may be gathered in June, dried, and made into tea. Be sure to cut away the stems before eating the flowers and remove the stems from berries too.

Wildlife/veterinary uses: At night raccoons raid this plant for the fruit. Numerous songbirds eat the berries. My tree is a favorite nesting site for a couple of prolific robins. Aphid infestations can wreck a tree.

Paper Birch, White Birch
Betula papyrifera Marsh.

Description: Brown-barked sapling matures into white-barked tree of medium height. Bark peeling, paperlike, separates into layers clearly marked with horizontal stripes. Twigs slightly rough, warty, odorless. Leaf buds blunt, hairless. Leaves heart shaped, 1 to 4 inches long. Fruiting catkins for flowers. Paper birch is also known as white birch.

Location: Across the northern tier of the United States, throughout Canada, and in the southern half of Alaska. Loamy to sandy well-drained soil; in and around lowland and alpine areas.

Food: White birch and yellow birch (*B. alleghaniensis*) may be tapped for their sap in late winter and early spring.

Traditional uses: White birch was considered by Native Americans and herbalists as a tonic and blood purifier. The bark powder was used on diaper rash and other skin rashes. The Cree Indians used the bark powder to treat chapping and venereal disease. The Ojibwas used it for stomach cramps. The outer bark was used as a poultice to cover wounds and as a cast for broken limbs. Wood was boiled in water and drunk to stimulate lactation. A decoction of the ends of stems and new growth treated toothache and teething. The inner bark was used in decoction for treating diarrhea. The decoction of new-growth tips of branches was used as a tea or tonic. Stomach cramps were treated with decocted root bark mixed with maple syrup. Sap was used to treat coughs.

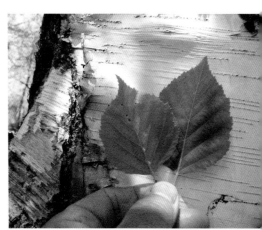

Paper birch, *Betula papyrifera*

Modern uses: Birch leaf extract is Commission E–approved for urinary tract infections, rheumatism, and bladder and kidney stones.

CAUTION: Birch leaf extract is not to be taken if you have edema, heart disease, or kidney dysfunction.

Notes: Shredded from the tree, the bark makes an excellent survival fire starter. The bone-dry, whitish wood from the top of a beaver dam is often the best source of firewood in the bush. Yellow birch, a long-lived species, has close-grained hardwood with rich dark tones and is used for tool handles, snowshoe frames, sleds, and sledges. The tough bark is peeled and stretched to make birch bark canoes. Canoe frames are made of white cedar and pine, and balsam resin is used to seal seams. Rotten birch wood is burned and used for smoking foods.

Wildlife/veterinary uses: Beavers eat the cambium beneath the bark, stripping the wood clean, and then use the wood to build dams and lodges. White birch leaves and end twigs are winter forage for moose, deer, and hare. Grouse and ptarmigan feed on the buds, and smaller birds and rodents eat the seeds.

Tamarack, American Larch
Larix laricina (Du Boi) K. Koch.

Description: Medium to large deciduous tree that at first glance looks like a pine or fir. Bark flakes off in scales. Nondrooping branchlets (in contrast, the European larch has drooping branches). Needles slender, to 1 inch long, in clusters, single or several, emanating from short spurs on branch. Cones less than ¾ inch long.

Location: Northern wetlands. The bald cypress is a similar species is found in wet areas of the southern United States.

Food: Tender new shoots can be infused into tea or pan-fried as food. The inner bark can be scraped, dried, and pounded into flour. Reconstitute it with water and make flatbread.

Traditional uses: Native Americans used a decoction of tamarack bark extraction in combination with balsam resin and other plants to treat acute infections such as colds, flu, fever, and coughs. Various tribes used the bark infusion of young shoots as a laxative. A bark and wood poultice was used to treat wounds and draw out infection. The inner bark infusion was considered warming. The resinous balsam was used as a stimulating inhalant. Leaf and bark were pounded, crushed, and used as a poultice to reduce headache. This ritual sweat lodge plant is useful for relieving tension, backache, and headache; its needles, twig, and bark were dampened and applied to hot stones to produce steam.

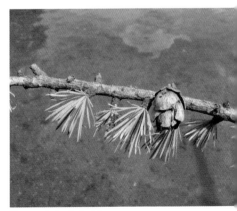

Tamarack, *Larix laricina*

Western larch, *L. occidentalis,* found west of the Plains states, was used in similar ways, including a decoction of the new growth as a wash for cancer. The resinous pitch of the western species was mixed with animal fat and used on wounds, cuts, and burns.

Modern uses: *L. decidua,* tamarack's European cousin, is Commission E–approved for coughs, colds, bronchitis, and fever and to promote resistance to acute infections. The outer bark extraction and balsam (resin) are used to make ointments, gels, and other emulsions for external application.

Notes: This rot-resistant relative of cypress makes long-lived railroad ties. The tree's tough, fibrous, and rot-resistant roots make good material for sewing and for weaving baskets, and it was often used to sew birch bark together to make canoes. The shredded inner bark was fed to horses.

Wildlife/veterinary uses: Needles, seeds, bark, and inner bark are eaten by grouse, snowshoe hare, porcupine, and squirrels. Seeds are eaten by nuthatches, chickadees, and crossbills.

Spirea: Hardhack Spirea; Subalpine Spirea
Spiraea douglasii Hook.; *S. densiflora*

Description: *S. douglasii* is an erect, many-branched perennial to 7 feet tall. Plants grow in thicket-sized colonies. Leaves alternate, oval to oblong; 2 to 6 inches long; dark green above, gray and woolly underneath. Rosy pink flowers, small and numerous, grow in a clublike

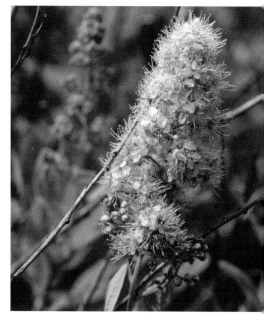

Spirea, *Spiraea douglasii*

terminal cluster that is longer than wide, whereas the flower cluster of *S. densiflora* is wider than tall. *S. densiflora* is typically about half as tall as *S. douglasii.*

Location: *S. douglasii* is found in western mountainous areas and coastal wet areas. Along stream banks, wetlands, lakeshores, damp meadows from sea level to mid elevations. *S. densiflora* is a subalpine member found on the slopes of Mount Baker and Mount Rainier and other mountains of the West.

Food: Aerial parts are decocted and taken as a health-protecting tea.

Traditional uses: The numerous spirea species were all used medicinally by Native Americans. The aerial parts contain an aspirin-like compound. Native Americans crushed the seeds and used them in tea to treat diarrhea. Aerial parts were infused as a tonic.

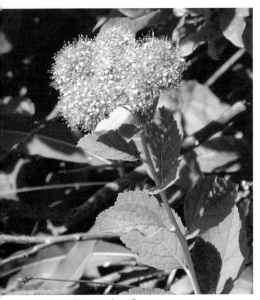

Spirea, *Spiraea densiflora*

Modern uses: Still used by some people in the traditional way. The aspirin-like compound collected in the tea may account for analgesic effect.

Notes: This attractive and tall wildflower is aggressive; so contain it along walls, shorelines, and fencerows. Its brushy stems were made into brooms by Native Americans.

Wildlife/veterinary uses: Dried flower spikes are eaten by wood grouse and ptarmigan.

Bees visit the flowers for pollen. One species is used in Germany as veterinary medicine in the much the same ways as the traditional human uses (see www.liberherbarum.com/Pn0805.htm).

CHAPTER 6

Medicinal Plants of the Mountain West

When the white men first came in, some of them tried to smoke the Indian tobacco. They thought: "We can smoke it." They took it into their lungs. Just once, they thought, "We will do like Indians do." Then they were sick for a week. The Indian tobacco is so strong.

—KARUK INFORMANT QUOTED BY HARRINGTON IN *BUREAU OF AMERICAN ETHNOLOGY BULLETIN* 91 (1929)

Western Skunk Cabbage

Lysichiton americanum Hultén and St. John

Description: Perennial with green to yellow elephant ear–like leaves, to 3 feet in length, lustrous and waxy in appearance, with skunky odor when torn. Yellow flower is an archaic, showy sheath surrounding a clublike flower spike.

Location: West of the Rocky Mountains north into British Columbia. Undercover in wet woods, swamps, lowlands, wet coastal areas.

Food: Never eat these plants fresh and uncooked. They contain toxic oxalate crystals that will burn your digestive system if eaten raw and fresh. Western skunk cabbage leaves and roots were washed and steamed or pit cooked until

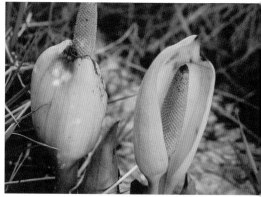

Western skunk cabbage, *Lysichiton americanum*

they reached a mushlike consistency. Several Western tribes ate roots after boiling them in eight changes of water. Root can be dried, roasted and ground into flour. Leaves were placed over cooking vegetables as a spice. Young leaves were thoroughly dried, then cooked in soups.

Drying the leaves or roots of Western skunk caggage eliminates some of the peppery, hot taste of the calcium oxalate crystals. The waxy leaves were used as plates for meals, to line cooking pits and cedar cooking boxes, to wrap meat and vegetables for pit-style cooking, and to store foods and cover fresh berries. Roots are numerous and tentacle-like.

Traditional uses: Western skunk cabbage was used in the same way as the smaller-leaved eastern skunk cabbage (*Symplocarpus foetidus*). Western skunk cabbage flowers were steamed and placed against joints to treat arthritis. Warm leaves were used in the sweat lodge as sitting mats to treat arthritis. A poultice of smashed root was used on boils and abscesses. The root was burned and its smoke inhaled to treat nightmares, disrupted sleep, and flu. The leaves served as poultice for burns. The Makah tribe chewed the raw root to induce abortion. Charcoal from the burned plants was applied to wounds. Steamed roots were used to treat arthritis.

Modern uses: A liquid extract of skunk cabbage is still used to treat bronchitis and asthma. The plant is considered antispasmodic, expectorant, sedative, and diaphoretic. Its use is reserved for skilled practitioners only.

CAUTION: Skunk cabbage contains poisonous oxalate crystals that will burn the digestive track if eaten raw and fresh. Only experts should use this plant.

Notes: Botanical Beach in Port Renfrew on Vancouver Island has some of the largest-leaved skunk cabbages I have ever seen. A small child could use one for a sleeping bag. The leaf veins are tough enough to make emergency cordage or sutures.

Wildlife/veterinary uses: Botanically, skunk cabbage is endothermic: It generates enough heat to melt snow and ice around its base. It comes up through the soil about a month before other plants.

False Hellebore
Veratrum viride Ait.

Description: Perennial that projects itself from the soil in spring, often in a colony of thick shoots, tubes of the rolled leaves. Basal leaves football shaped, with deep veins; to 12 inches, leaves smaller as they unfurl up the single 3-foot-tall unbranched central stalk. Flowers yellow to green, born on branching terminal stalks at top of plant. Fruit to 1½ inches in length, containing winged seeds.

Location: The mountainous West.

Food: False hellebore shoots look edible, but are toxic. Blackfoot Indians ingested the plant to commit suicide.

Traditional uses: A poultice of the bulb was used to treat arthritis. The Bella Coolas took a bulb decoction for respiratory problems such as chronic cough. The raw root and decoction were considered emetic. The Blackfoot peoples dried and powdered the root to use it like snuff as an analgesic for headaches. Snuffing the powder also induced sneezing. The Cowlitz placed poulticed leaves over painful areas.

Modern uses: False hellebore is an obsolete drug. Its steroid saponins are severely toxic, and the inherent toxic alkaloids stimulate motor neurons, leading to convulsions and respiratory failure.

CAUTION: Toxic! Look but don't touch.

Notes: False hellebore, one of the most striking plants of the mountainous West, was integral to Spanish traditional medicine. *V. album* root, a close relative of *V. viride,* was used as an analgesic, emetic, cathartic, antirrheumatic, and sternutatory (induces sneezing). The root was prepared with oil or grease as a salve. Once reserved for the skilled holistic health-care provider, today false hellebore is considered too toxic to warrant further use.

Wildlife/veterinary uses: The false hellebore *V. californicum* of California was used by the Paiutes as a snakebite remedy. A poultice of pulped root was applied to snakebites. They also applied the poultice over saddle sores on horses.

Arnica
Arnica spp.: *A. montana* L.; *A. acaulis* Walt; *A. cordifolia* Hook; *A. latifolia* Bong.

Description: Perennial to 18 inches. Rhizome brownish. Leaves form a basal rosette. Hairy stem rises from the rosette and has two to six smaller leaves, ovate to lance shaped and dentate (toothed). Terminal yellow flowers emerge from the axil of the top pair of leaves. Flowers are from 2 to 3 inches in diameter with hairy receptacle and hairy calyx. Tiny disk

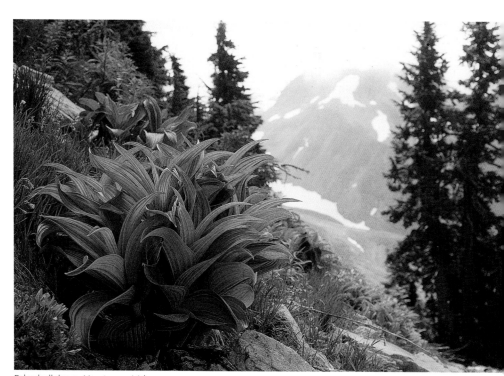

False hellebore, *Veratrum viride*

flowers reside inside the corolla and are tubular; as many as 100 disk flowers per flower head.

Location: Typically shady mountainous areas, along seeps and stream banks to 10,000 feet, and wet alpine meadows.

Food: Not edible; toxic. Internal consumption causes stomach pain, vomiting, and diarrhea. High doses may induce cardiac arrest.

Traditional uses: Volatile oils in the flowers were used in making perfume. Native Americans used an infusion of the roots externally for back pain. A poultice was used on edemas to reduce swelling. The plant was considered anthelminthic, antiseptic, astringent, choleretic, emmenagogue, expectorant, febrifuge, stimulant, and tonic. Typically it was used as a topical agent for wound healing. The whole plant used after extraction in ointment or as a compress with antimicrobial and fungicidal action. In folk medicine it was used to induce abortions.

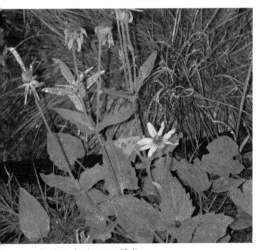

Arnica, *Arnica cordifolia*

Modern uses: Commission E–approved for treating fevers, colds, coughs, bronchitis, skin inflammations, mouth and pharynx inflammations, rheumatism, injuries, and tendencies toward infection (weakened immunity). Medicinal parts include the roots and rhizome, dried flowers, and leaves collected before flowering. Because of the toxic nature of the plant, homeopathic doses are used to manage pain, to treat diabetic retinopathy, and to treat muscle soreness. The plant extract is used in antidandruff preparations and hair tonics. In clinical research arnica has presented mixed results as an anti-inflammatory.

CAUTION: Flowers may be a skin irritant, causing eczema. Do not use during pregnancy. Do not use if sensitive (allergic) to members of the daisy family. Health-care practitioners are warned not to use arnica on mucous membranes, open skin wounds, or the eyes. Do not use orally except in homeopathic concentrations. Arnica may interact with anticoagulants and induce bleeding.

Notes: Arnica species are abundant in the mountainous West from the Little Bighorns through the Rockies and on into the Pacific Northwest. They are numerous in and around the slopes of Mount Rainier, Mount Adams, and Mount Baker in the Cascades of Washington state.

Wildlife/veterinary uses: Arnica is an important food for song and game birds and ground cover for small game. Native Americans used juniper branches around tepees and shelters to fend off rattlesnakes. Arnica is used with horses to treat aches and pains.

Sitka Valerian
Valeriana sitchensis Bong.; *V. officinalis*

Description: Perennial to 24 inches, sometimes higher. Leaves opposite, staggered up the stem, often with several basal leaves. Terminal cluster of white- to cream-colored odiferous flowers, petals are feathery. Blooms April to July.

Location: Montane plant, typically found on north-facing slopes. Plentiful in alpine meadows and along trails in the Olympics, Cascades, North Cascades, Mount Rainier, and Mount Baker, especially along Heliotrope Trail toward the climbers' route.

Food: Edible roots are not worth the effort. (If you have had the foul-smelling valerian tea, you are nodding your head in agreement.)

Traditional uses: Stress-reducing, tension-relieving mild sedative for insomniacs. *V. sitchensis* roots were decocted in water to treat pain, colds, and diarrhea. A poultice of the root was used to treat cuts, wounds, bruises, and inflammation.

Modern uses: A few people still use *V. sitchensis* in the traditional way. Aqueous extract of *V. officinalis* root in a double-blind study had significant effect on poor or irregular sleepers, smokers. Sometimes combined with hops (*Humulus lupulus*) and skullcap (*Scutellaria lateriflora*). The effect of valerian on gamma amino butyric acid (GABA) may reduce blood pressure and help mild depression. This chemical is also found in evening primrose seeds and several varieties of tomatoes.

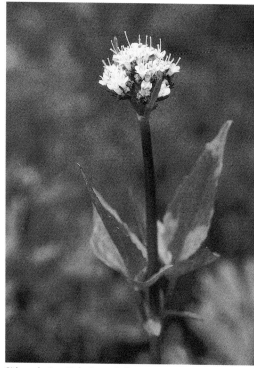

Sitka valerian, *Valeriana sitchensis*

Notes: Take the road to the Sunrise Lodge on the northside of Mount Rainier, walk to the learning-center garden, and see this plant and many other medicinal plants of the West and Northwest. A splendid setting. The plant's odiferous flowers are not particularly pleasant to many, but I love that stink; it means I'm back in the mountains.

Wildlife/veterinary uses: One might try using root extract, as is done with other valerians, as bait to lure wild cats, rodents, and mountain lions in close for hair-raising photo opportunities. Deer forage on the leaves of this plant. *V. edulis* extract is used in animal calming products such as Ultra Calm, and as part of a fertility booster for horses.

Bistort, Meadow Bistort; Alpine Bistort

Polygonum bistortoides Pursh.;
P. viviparum L.

Description: Perennial to 30 inches. Basal leaves. White flowers in single dense cluster atop erect stalk, later forming a seed head with brownish achenes (seeds).

Location: Both species grow from New Mexico to Alaska on wet, open slopes. Abundant in the alpine meadows of Mount Rainier and the Cascades.

Food: Young leaves and shoots are edible raw or cooked. They have a slightly sour taste. Older leaves are tough and stringy. Use leaves in salads and cooked with meat. The starchy root is edible boiled in soups and stews or soaked in water, dried, and ground into flour for biscuits, rolls, and bread. The cooked roots are said to taste like almonds or chest-nuts. The seeds are edible and pleasant tasting.

Traditional uses: This vitamin C–rich plant was used to treat or prevent scurvy. As an alcohol tincture it is astringent and used externally on cuts, abrasions, acne, insect stings and bites, inflammations, and infections.

Modern uses: Little used today as a medicinal. Traditional uses still employed by montane-dwelling Native Americans and Europeans.

Notes: Easily identified and harvested in areas where harvesting is allowed.

Wildlife/veterinary uses: Flowers of *P. amphibium* are used as fish bait.

Beargrass

Xerophyllum tenax (Pursh) Nutt.

Description: Perennial to 3 feet in height. A stout grass with sharp, long, saw-edged blades, blue green in color, producing a long, central flower stalk with terminal raceme crowded with white flowers. A distinctive plant, no look-alikes; once you see it you'll never forget.

Location: Mountainous West north from California to Alaska, east to Montana and Wyoming. Mountain slopes, openings in alpine forests, edges of mountain lakes and streams to the tree line.

Food: Roots can be boiled until tender and eaten.

Traditional uses: According to Moerman (*Native American Ethnobotany;* appendix D), Blackfoot Indians chewed the roots and applied them to wounds as

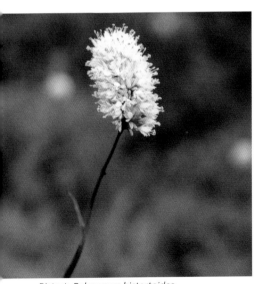
Bistort, *Polygonum bistortoides*

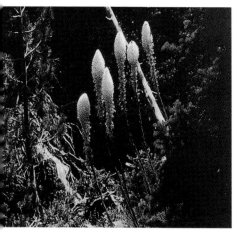

Beargrass, *Xerophyllum tenax*

a poultice. Pounded and grated roots were applied externally to sprains and broken bones. Other indigenous folks used wet roots to wash wounds.

Modern uses: No documented modern uses.

Notes: This plant is considered an environmental "canary in the mine": When beargrass disappears from a forest, the forest is in decline. Leaves are gathered for flower arranging. The tough leaves were used to decorate belts and dresses and to make baskets. Soaking the first leaves of spring softens them and makes the shoots pliable weaving material. The best stand of beargrass I ever saw was in Idaho along U.S. Highway 287 in the Beaverhead National Forest en route to the Bitterroots.

Wildlife/veterinary uses: According to Stewart (*Wildflowers of the Olympics and Cascades*), bears eat the roots. I have not found this documented anywhere else.

Usnea, Old Man's Beard
Usnea spp.

Description: Parasitic epiphyte, a tree lichen. There are numerous of hairlike parasitic organisms hanging from conifers. Usnea is light gray green and best identified by teasing apart the outer mycelia sheath of its skin to expose a tough white central core or cord, thread-like and supple. Other clinging lichens do not have this white central core.

Location: Forests of the Pacific Northwest and in the broader north temperate climate zone; worldwide in moist and damp habitats.

Food: Unlike other lichen species, usnea is not eaten.

Traditional uses: Native Americans moistened the crushed plant and applied it as a poultice over boils and wounds. In traditional Chinese medicine it is used to treat tuberculosis. In Europe and Asia it was used for thousands of years as an anti-infective.

Modern uses: Commission E–approved for mouth inflammations and inflammations of the pharynx. Widely used by naturopaths to treat acute bacterial and fungal infections. Scientific studies report that the extract is effective against gram-positive bacteria (pneumococcus and streptococcus). Antiviral effects have been shown in vitro. Where available, the drug is produced in the form of lozenges.

Notes: Campers used the lichen as stuffing material for mattresses, pillows, as a soft bedding under sleeping bag. Moerman (*Native American Ethnobotany*)

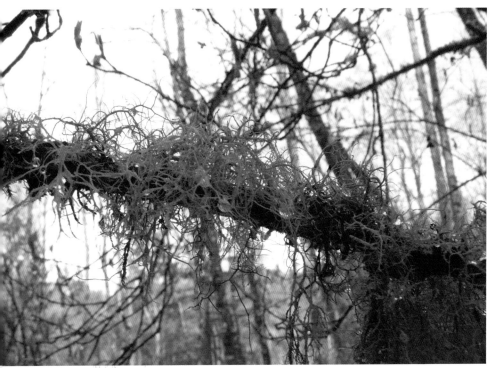

Usnea, *Usnea* sp.

reports that the Nitinaht women used usnea as sanitary napkins and as diaper material for babies.

Wildlife/veterinary uses: Nesting material for birds.

Arrowleaf Balsam Root

Balsamorhiza sagittata (Pursh) Nutt.

Description: There are numerous species. *B. sagittata* grows 1 to 2 feet in height and is found in clumps. Leaves basal, petioled, and arrow shaped; hairy, rough to the touch; from 8 to 12 inches in length. Flowers yellow, long stalked. Up to twenty-two yellow rays encircle the yellow disc of florets.

Location: Foothills and higher elevation of the Rockies from Colorado to British Columbia. Dry, sunny slopes.

Food: Young leaves and shoots are edible, as well as young flower stalks and young stems. They may be steamed or eaten raw. Peeled roots are also eaten but are bitter unless slow-cooked to break down the indigestible polysaccharide (inulin). The roots may be cooked and dried, then reconstituted in simmering water before eating. Seeds are eaten out of hand or pounded into a meal used as flour. The roasted seeds can be ground into pinole. The Nez Perce roasted and ground the seeds, which they then formed into little balls by adding grease.

Traditional uses: Native Americans used the wet leaves as a wound dressing and a poultice over burns. The sticky sap sealed wounds and was considered antiseptic. Although balsam root is bitter when peeled and chewed, it contains inulin that may stimulate the immune system, providing protection from acute sickness such as colds and flu. The sap is considered antibacterial and antifungal. A decoction of the leaves, stems, and roots was taken for stomachache and colds. The root was also used for treating gonorrhea and syphilis. In the sweat lodge, balsam root smoke and steam is reported to relieve headaches. It is considered a warrior plant, and in smudging ceremonies it is a disinfectant and inhaled for body aches. The chewed root was used as a poultice over sores, wounds, and burns.

Modern uses: Little studied or used in any modern context. Traditional uses are still practiced.

Notes: This plant is widespread in the Bitterroots and other Idaho wilderness areas. In a pinch—should you get lost in these vast mountainous expanses—here is a food that helps you survive. But freeing the root, often deeply and intricately woven into the rock, is an exhausting task.

Wildlife/veterinary uses: A poultice of the root is used on saddle sores. It is low-quality forage for lamb, often used to test discriminating prowess of lambs when arrowleaf is coupled with a better forage. Leaves are eaten by Rocky Mountain elk, mule deer, pronghorn antelope, bighorn sheep, and Columbia ground squirrels.

Pipsissewa
Chimaphila umbellata (L.) Nutt.

Description: Small evergreen shrub to 12 inches in height. Glossy green leaves in whorls, lance-shaped, shiny, toothed. Whitish pink to rose-colored flowers, about ⅜ inch across, grow in clusters atop a long stem. Fruit is round.

Location: Nationwide in forests, foothills, and montane coniferous woods of Colorado, Wyoming, Montana, Alberta, and British Columbia south to California and east to Maine, south to Florida. Not found in the American Southwest, Kentucky, or Tennessee.

Food: The plant is used as a flavoring agent for candy and pop, and the leaves and roots are boiled and eaten. Berries are eaten as a digestive.

Traditional uses: The tea was used as an expectorant considered a dermatological, urinary, and orthopedic aid. Tea made from aerial parts was used to treat water retention and kidney and bladder problems. An infusion from the plant was

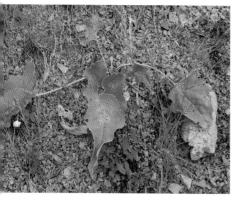
Arrowleaf balsam root, *Balsamorhiza sagittata*

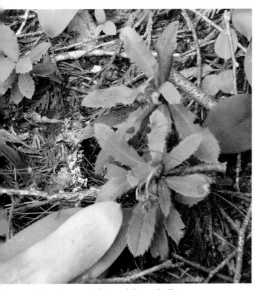

Pipsissewa , *Chimaphila umbellata*

Modern uses: Considered to be a treatment for kidney problems. Used by homeopathic practitioners to treat inflammation of urinary tract, mammary glands, and prostrate.

CAUTION: Leaves applied as a poultice may cause inflammation and dermatitis.

Notes: This fragrant flower grows in profusion around the slopes of Mount Baker and Mount Rainier in Washington State, but it has been overharvested and is becoming difficult to find elsewhere.

Wildlife/veterinary uses: An infusion of the leaves was used in veterinary medicine for the diseases of horses. See more at www.geocities.com/littleflowers_medicinal_plants/pipsissewa.htm. For a cat with a kidney problem, see your vet and ask about using a decoction of parsley, pipsissewa, juniper, and goldenrod. For more information go to www.herbnet.com and search "pipsissewa." The plant is used in farm animals in the same way it was traditionally used in humans.

used as an eyewash. The astringent herb was used to treat fevers, stomachaches, backaches, coughs, and sore throats and as a wash for wounds, sores, blisters, and rashes. Fresh leaves were crushed and applied externally to reduce inflammation. Native Americans used the tea to regulate menstruation.

*In this silent, serene wilderness the weary can gain
a heart-bath in perfect peace.*

—JOHN MUIR

Devil's Club
Oplopanax horridus Sm.
Torr. & Gray ex Miq

Description: Shrubby perennial to 10
feet. Spreading, crooked, and tangled
growth covered with horrible thorns.
Wood has sweet odor. Dinner-plate-size
maplelike leaves with seven to nine
sharp-pointed leaves armed underneath
with thorns. Clublike flower head with
white flowers grouped in a compact ter-

minal head. Berries shiny bright red,
flattened.

Location: Coastal mountains and coast-
line. Seepage sites, stream banks, moist
low-lying forested areas, old avalanche
tracks. Typically grows at low altitude, but
in Canada it may grow to the tree line.

Food: Not often eaten as food, its berries
are considered inedible. According to
Moerman (*Native American Ethnobotany;*
see appendix D), spring buds were boiled
and eaten by the Oweekeno tribe.

Traditional uses: Related to ginseng,
devil's club's roots, berries, and especially
greenish inner bark are used. The plant is
one of the most important medicinal
plants of West Coast First Peoples and is
still used in rituals and medicine. Berries
are rubbed into hair to kill lice or shine
hair. The inner bark is chewed raw as a
purgative and emetic or taken with hot
water for the same purpose. The inner
bark is infused or decocted to treat stomach and bowel cramps, arthritis, stomach
ulcers, and other unspecified illnesses of

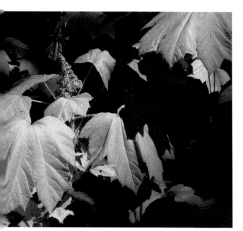

Devil's club, *Oplopanax horridus*

127

the digestive system. Root, leaves, and stems are added to hot baths and sweat lodges to treat arthritis. The cooked and shredded root bark is used as a poultice for many skin conditions. The stem decoction is used for reducing fever. Tea from the inner bark is used for treating diabetes, a common ailment in aboriginal people who now eat a fatty and carbohydrate-rich Western diet. The dried root was mixed with tobacco and smoked to treat headache. An infusion of crushed stems was used as a blood purifier. Stem ashes and oil were used on skin ailments. The traditional use as an abortifacient has been disproved.

Modern uses: The plant continues to be used by Native Americans in traditional ways. German clinical trials show the plant has anti-inflammatory and analgesic activity. Animal studies show that a methanolic extract of the roots reduces blood pressure and heart rate (see Circosta et al., "Cardiovascular Activity," part 2, *Journal of Ethnopharmocology* 72 [1994]: 1532).

Notes: Native Americans burned devil's club, then mixed the ashes with grease to make a black face paint that was said to give a warrior supernatural power. Bella Coola Indians used the spiny sticks as protective charms. The scraped bark was boiled with grease to make dye. Native Americans hunters sponge a decoction of the plant's bark over their body to remove human odor.

Wildlife/veterinary uses: Northwest tribes carved fishing lures from the thorny wood.

Red Alder
Alnus rubra Bong.

Description: Member of the birch family to 80 feet in height, often much smaller. Bark smooth and gray when young, coarse and whitish gray when mature. *A. rubra* bark turns red to orange when exposed to moisture. Leaves are bright green, oval, coarsely toothed and pointed. Male flowers clustered in long hanging catkins; female seed capsule is ovoid cone. Seed nuts small, slightly winged, flat.

Location: Species ranges from California to Alaska east to Idaho. Moist areas.

Food: Members of this genus provide a generous resource of firewood in the Northwest for savory barbecue cooking. The bark and wood chips are preferred over mesquite for smoking fish, especially salmon. The sweet inner bark is scraped in the early spring and eaten fresh, raw, or combined with flour to make cakes.

Traditional uses: Sweat-lodge floors were often covered in alder leaf, and switches of alder were used for applying water to the body and the hot rocks. Alder ashes were used as a paste with a chewing stick to clean the teeth. Cones of subspecies *A. sinuata* are also used for medicine, as are other alder species. Spring catkins were smashed to pulp and eaten as a cathartic (to help move the bowels). The bark was sometimes mixed with other plants in decoction and used as a tonic. Female catkins were used in decoction to treat gonorrhea. A poultice of leaves was applied to skin wounds and

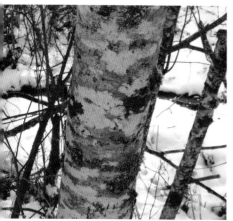
Red alder, *Alnus rubra*

skin infections. In the Okanagan area of central Washington and British Columbia, First Peoples used an infusion of new end shoots as an appetite stimulant for children. The leaf tea infusion said to be an itch- and inflammation-relieving wash for insect bites and stings and poison ivy and poison oak. Upper Tanana informants reported that a decoction of the inner bark reduces fever. An infusion of bark was used to wash sores, cuts, and wounds.

Modern uses: This is still an important warrior plant in sweat lodge ceremonies. For more on sweat lodges, see the DVD *Native American Medicine* (appendix D). Black alder, *A. glutinosa,* is endemic to the Northern Hemisphere and is used in Russia and former Eastern Block countries as a gargle to relieve sore throat and reduce fever. Research suggest that betulin and lupeol in alder may inhibit tumor growth.

Notes: To smoke meat with alder, soak the wood chips overnight in water, then place the moist chips on coals or char-

coal to smoke meat. In 1961 I saw more than a hundred Native Americans smoking fish, moose, and caribou for winter storage along a 10-mile stretch of the Denali Highway in Alaska. Hunting rules at that time required any person shooting a caribou to give some of the meat to the First Peoples, who preserved it for winter food. Fish were flayed, stabbed through with a stick, and hung from wood weirs above a smoldering alder fire until smoked and dry. Ashes of alder were mixed with tobacco and smoked. In hardwood-poor areas of the West, alder burns slower than pine and is a suitable home heating fuel. Bark may be stripped and soaked in water to make an orange-to-rust dye. Numerous alder species are found across North America, often in impenetrable mazes surrounding stream beds—great bear habitat, so be careful.

Wildlife/veterinary uses: The reddish brown bark dye makes fishnets invisible to fish. Wood is carved to make fishing arrow points.

Western Red Cedar
Thuja plicata D. Don.

Description: Aromatic evergreen to 75 feet in height. Many branched from the trunk skyward. Needles flattened; dark green above, lighter green below. Heavy seed crops are produced every three years. Fertility is reached at about twenty years of age.

Location: Windward side of the Cascades, including Vancouver Island and the Olympic Peninsula. Moist bottomland with deep rich soils.

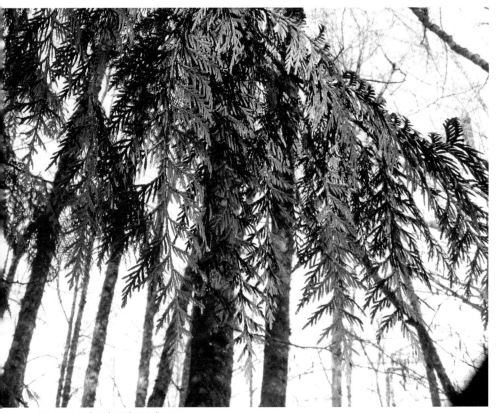

Western red cedar, *Thuja plicata*

Food: *T. plicata*'s primary use is and was for making cooking boxes and planks for flavoring and cooking salmon. The cambium (inner bark) could be eaten as a survival food, but there are numerous other safer alternatives (see Meuninck, *Basic Essentials Edible Wild Plants;* appendix D).

Traditional uses: *T. plicata,* red cedar, is a male warrior plant used by Native Americans in sweeping and smudging and steam bath rituals to clear the body and mind of evil spirits that prevent good health. Northwestern tribes make fine cedar boxes for cooking and storage. Europeans use the wood to line chests and encasements because of the fine fragrance and insect-repelling chemistry of the wood. A decoction of dried and powdered leaves was used as an external analgesic to treat painful joints, sores, wounds, and injuries. Leaves in infusion were used to treat coughs and colds. The decoction of the bark in water was used to induce menstruation and possibly as an abortifacient. The leaf buds (new end growth) were chewed to treat lung ailments. A decoction of leaves and boughs was used to treat arthritis.

Modern uses: *T. occidentalis* is preferred over *T. plicata* as a homeopathic drug to treat rheumatism, poor digestion, depression, and skin conditions.

CAUTION: Because of its thujone content, this is a drug that must be used with professional consultation and supervision.

Notes: This magnificent tree, tall and thick, is a giant of old-growth forests in the Northwest. It makes a durable, decay-resistant wood. Cedar boxes are still used to steam salmon and other foods. Hot rocks are placed on wet plants—often skunk cabbage leaves—wrapped around the salmon. The box is covered with a lid and the salmon slow cooked in steam. Cedar boxes are also used for making seaweed more palatable. Red laver seaweed, *Porphyra perforata*, is decomposed for five days, then pressed into wood frames and dried in the sun, then transferred to cedar boxes. Then people chew chiton meat (from a tidal mollusk with an armorlike scaly shell) and spit the meat between layers of seaweed. The boxes are secured for about a month and then the ritual preparation is repeated three more times. Finally, the cakes are packed in a cedar box with cedar boughs and used as winter food, often eaten with salmon at potlatchlike feasts. The trunk of red cedar is used to make totem poles and canoes. The inner bark is used to make baskets.

Wildlife/veterinary uses: Red squirrels eat the buds in spring and cut and store seed-laden branches for winter forage. Rabbits, moose, and deer browse on the leaves. Porcupines eat the bark and may inadvertently girdle a tree, killing it. Boughs are used as a snake repellent.

Douglas Fir
Pseudotsuga menziesii (Mirbel) Franco

Description: Medium to large conifer; coastal variety grows to 240 feet. Narrow, pointed crown, slightly drooping branches, and straight trunk. Deeply furrowed bark on mature tree. Needles single, flat, pointed but soft ended, about 1 inch long, evenly spaced along the twigs. Cones to 4 inches long have winged seeds, three pointed bracts extending beyond cone scales look like the legs and rear end of a mouse hiding in the cone; distinctive.

Location: Mountainous West and West Coast, from Mexico north to British Columbia. Grows best on wet, well-drained slopes.

Food: The new end growth is made into a tea. The pitch is chewed like gum as a breath cleanser. Needles and branches are cooked with meat as flavoring. Rare Douglas fir sugar, or wild sugar, accumulates on the ends of branch tips on trees

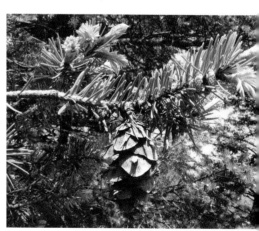

Douglas fir, *Pseudotsuga menziesii*

found in sunny exposures on midsummer days. According Harriet V. Kuhnlein and Nancy J. Turner (*Traditional Plant Foods of Canadian Indigenous Peoples*), the sugar candy looks like whitish, frostlike globules.

Traditional uses: This is a popular and important sweat-lodge plant. Its aromatic needled branches are steamed to treat rheumatism and in cleansing purification rituals. Buds, bark, leaves, new-growth end sprouts, and pitch are all used as medicine by Native Americans. A decoction of buds is unproven treatment for venereal diseases. The bark infusion was taken to treat bowel and stomach problems. The bark was burned and taken with water to treat diarrhea. The needle infusion was drunk to relieve paralysis. Leaves were made into tea to treat arthritic complaints. Pitch was used to seal wounds, chewed like gum to treat sore throat, and considered an effective first aid for cuts, abrasions, bites, and stings. Decoction of new-growth twigs, shoots, needles treated colds. Ashes of twigs and bark were mixed with fat to treat rheumatic arthritis.

Modern uses: Still very important ritual plant in Native American spiritual rites.

Notes: Excellent open firewood for cooking fish and meat. Also serves as an attractive Christmas tree and a top-ranked lumber tree, used to veneer plywood.

Wildlife/veterinary uses: The wood was used by Native Americans to make harpoon shafts, carved fish baits, wooden hooks, herring rakes, and wooden fish traps. Needle boughs were roughed over hunters to provide a fragrance that would disguise human odor.

Juniper
Juniperus communis L.

Description: Evergreen tree or low-lying spreading shrub; often grows in colonies. Leaves evergreen, pointy, stiff, somewhat flattened, light green; whorls of three spreading from the branches. Buds covered with scalelike needles. Berries blue, hard, emit a tangy smell when scraped, and impart a tangy flavor—a creosote-like taste. Male flowers are catkinlike with numerous stamens in three segmented whorls; female flowers are green and oval.

Location: Nationwide.

Food: Dried berries are cooked with game and fowl. Try putting them in a pepper mill and grating them into bean soup and stews and on wild game and domestic foul. The berries may be made into tea—simply crush one or two berries and add them to water just off the boil. Gin, vodka, schnapps, and aquavit are flavored with juniper berries. Use berries in grilling marinades. Grate berries on cold cuts and on vegetated protein cold cuts, like Wham and Gardenburgers. Be judicious; large amounts of the berry may be toxic (as are large amounts of pepper and salt), so use in small amounts like a spice.

Traditional uses: The diluted essential oil is applied to the skin to draw and cleanse deeper skin tissue. It has been used to promote menstruation and to relieve PMS and dysmenorrhea. Traditional practitioners use 1 teaspoon of participants. Mice trials suggest the berry extract in pharmaceutical doses to be anti-inflammatory, at least in the rodents. Juniper oil has been used successfully as a diuretic and may be useful as adjunct therapy for diabetes.

CAUTION: Use juniper sparingly, as allergic reactions are possible. Pregnant women should avoid this herb because it may induce uterine contractions. It may increase menstrual bleeding. Do not use if kidney infection or kidney disease is suspected. Do not use the concentrated and caustic essential oil internally without guidance from a licensed holistic healthcare practitioner.

Notes: I occasionally chew on a berry—ripe, soft ones are tastiest. Add a half-dozen berries to duck, goose, lamb, or goat stew and heighten the flavor adventure. Juniper is easily transplanted to your garden.

Wildlife/veterinary uses: A proprietary formula also contains yucca and reportedly helps repair and support joints in horses—search "Joint Support horses." Juniper is used in many of the traditional ways with pets; talk to your vet.

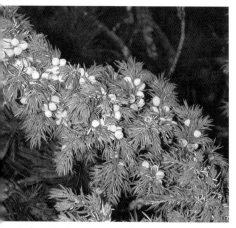

Juniper, *Juniperus communis*

berries to 1 cup of water, boil for three minutes, let steep until cool. A few practitioners add bark and needles to the berry tea. The berry is considered an antiseptic, a diuretic, a tonic, and a digestive aid. It's strongly antiseptic to urinary tract problems and gallbladder complaints but contraindicated in the presence of kidney disease.

Modern uses: Commission E–approved for treating dyspepsia. The berry is diuretic, so the extract is diuretic (Odrinil). It's possibly indicated for treating heart disease, high blood pressure, and dropsy. The berry extract is used in Europe to treat arthritis and gout. Animal studies of the extract in various combinations showed anti-inflammatory and anti-cancer activity, but this is not proven in humans. It decreased glycemic levels in diabetic rats. In human trials the berry extract combined with nettle and yarrow extracts failed to prevent gingivitis. In one double-blind, placebo-controlled study, juniper oil and wintergreen oil (30 milliliters of Kneipp-Rheumabad) were added to bath water and reduced pain in trial

Western Hemlock
Tsuga heterophylla (Raf.) Sarg.

Description: Evergreen to 150 feet in height. Narrow, conical crown. Slightly drooping branches. Needles spreading in two rows, to ¾ inch in length; flat, flexible, and rounded at the tip with a very short stalk—green above and whitish below, underside may have tiny teeth. Slender, brownish yellow twigs with fine hair, rough to the touch. Cones elliptical, long, brown, without a stalk, hanging down at the end of the twigs. Seeds paired and long winged.

Location: California north to southern Alaska and east to northern Idaho and Montana. Acid soils; moist, low flats; and lower slopes in dense stands.

Food: Inner bark is made into bread by coastal First Peoples.

Traditional uses: The outer bark was decocted and the wash was used to treat wounds and burns. The inner bark was scraped and infused to treat acute infections such as flu and colds. The oil and resin of hemlock was used externally as a rub to treat arthritis and rheumatic joints. Needle tea is antiscorbutic (high in vitamin C) and was used to prevent scurvy.

Modern uses: Teas and bark decoctions are still used in moderation by First Peoples. Herring eggs, an important food of northwestern First Peoples, are still harvested using hemlock boughs (see the notes). Modern pharmaceutical uses of hemlock are unproven and little employed.

CAUTION: Needle tea is occasionally taken for colds and flu, but it can be toxic in large amounts.

Notes: Hemlock makes excellent pulpwood and is a source of alpha cellulose used in manufacturing plastics, cellophane paper, and rayon. Native Americans made fishing lures, paddles, and boats from the wood and used the resinous pitch to waterproof boat seams and baskets. Boughs make excellent aromatic bedding when camping. Live trees are cut across streams by Native Americans to provide attachment places for herring spawn. The spawn-laden needles are harvesting and the spawn removed, prepared, and eaten. Hemlock wood is used to make sugar and flour barrels.

Wildlife/veterinary uses: This evergreen is an excellent food source for deer and elk and a nesting site for bald eagles. Trappers used the boughs, wood, and bark to boil traps to remove human odor, and boughs were used to collect herring spawn. Saplings were stripped of boughs and twigs and then used as poles for salmon dip nets. Knots of the tree are dense and tough and were carved to make fishhooks. Animal and fish traps are made from the boughs.

Madrone
Arbutus menziesii Pursh.

Description: Evergreen, broadleaf tree to 100 feet in height. Young bark chartreuse and smooth; older bark dark brown to red, peeling. Evergreen leaves alternate, oval, 7 inches long, shiny; dark green above, lighter, whitish green beneath;

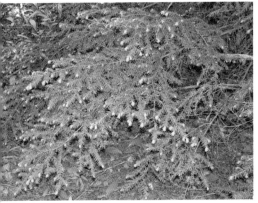
Western hemlock, *Tsuga heterophylla*

hairless and leathery. White flowers urn shaped, to 3 inches long, in large drooping clusters. Berry orange red, about ½ inch across, with granular skin.

Location: Coastal areas of northern California, Oregon, Washington, and British Columbia. Dry, sunny areas with a sea exposure.

Food: People of the Vancouver Salish nation used the reddish bark in decoction to dye the white edible camas bulbs pink. Berries have been eaten, but there's little documentation. Berries were cooked before eating or were steamed, dried, and stored and then reconstituted in hot water before eating. Berries were also smashed and made into a ciderlike drink. The Miwoks claimed the cider was an appetite stimulant and it resolved upset stomach.

Traditional uses: The Saanich and other Indian nations used bark and leaves for treating colds, tuberculosis, and stomach problems and as a postpartum contraceptive. Decoctions of the plant were also used as an emetic. Leaves were used by Cowichans of the Northwest as a burn treatment and wound dressing. The leaf infusion was used to treat stomach ulcers, and leaves were eaten off the tree to relieve cramps. The juice from the chewed leaves reportedly relieved sore throat. A leaf infusion was used by the Skokomish people to treat colds and treat ulcers. A bark infusion was used to treat diarrhea. An astringent bark decoction was used for washing sores, wounds, and impetigo and as a gargle for sore throat, according to Pomo and Kashaya people. The Karoks used leaves in their puberty ceremony.

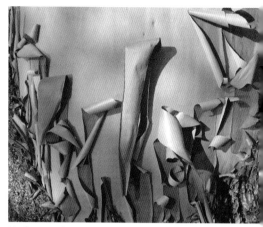
Madrone, *Arbutus menziesii*

Modern uses: No longer studied.

Notes: This is perhaps my favorite tree of the Northwest. The wood was used to make canoes. Berries were also dried and used as beads when making bracelets and necklaces.

Wildlife/veterinary uses: Livestock eat the flowers, as do many wild animals. Leaves are eaten by cows. An infusion of leaves and bark was used by Native Americans to relieve sore muscles in horses. The berries serve as steelhead trout bait.

Oregon Grape
Mahonia aquifolium (Pursh) Nutt.;
M. nervosa (Pursh) Nutt. var. *nervosa*

Description: *M. aquifolium*: Evergreen shrub to 6 feet tall. Gray stem. Hollylike, shiny leaves; pinnate, compound, pointed edges. Flower small, bright yellow. Berries deep blue, waxy. Roots and root hairs, when peeled, are bright yellow inside due to the alkaloid berberine. *M. nervosa* is a smaller forest dweller with

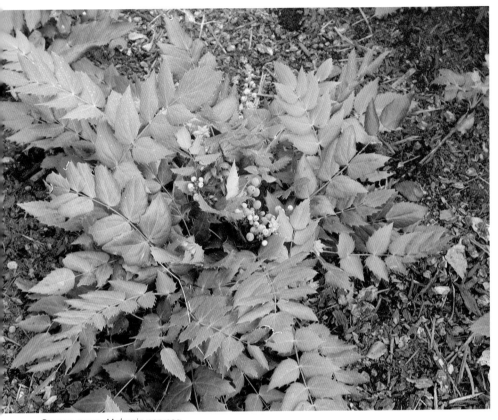

Oregon grape, *Mahonia nervosa*

rosette of compound leaves in a whorl up to 3 feet tall, berries on central spikes.

Location: *M. aquifolium*: Washington State east into Idaho and Montana. Along roadsides and forest edges. *M. nervosa*: Pacific Northwest. Along Mount Baker Highway in Washington en route to Mount Baker, in open forests and grave-yards.

Food: The tart berries of *M. aquifolium* are eaten in late summer in Northwest. Native Americans smashed the berries and dried them for later use. They may be boiled into jam, but be certain to add honey or sugar, because the juice is tart. Carrier Indians of the Northwest sim-

mered the young leaves and ate them. The smaller creeping *M. nervosa* was pre-pared and eaten in the same way and is preferred, but it is not as abundant. Try berries mixed with other fruit to improve the taste. Berries may be pounded into paste, formed into cakes, and dried for winter food.

Traditional uses: When eaten raw in small amounts, the fruit is slightly emetic. Tart berries of both species were consid-ered a morning-after pick-me-up. Native Americans believed the berries were slightly emetic. A decoction of stems was used by Sanpoils as an antiemetic. These two species of bitter and astringent herbs were used to treat liver and gallbladder complaints. The bark infusion was used by Native Americans as an eyewash. According to traditional use, the decocted drug from the inner bark (berberine) stimulates the liver and gallbladder, cleansing them, releasing toxins, and increasing the flow of bile. The bark and root decoction reportedly was used externally for treating *staphylococcus* infections. According to Michael Moore (*Medicinal Plants of the Mountain West*), the drug stimulates thyroid function and is used to treat diarrhea and gastritis. According to Deni Brown (*Encyclopedia of Herbs and Their Uses*), *M. aquifolium* has been used to treat chronic hepatitis and dry-type eczema. A root decoction of *M. aquifolium* was used by the Blackfoot peoples to stem hemorrhaging. They also used roots in decoction for upset stomach and to treat other stomach problems.

Modern uses: *M. aquifolium* extractions are available in commercial ointments to treat dry skin, unspecified rashes, and psoriasis. The bitter drug may prove an appetite stimulant, but little research has been done. Other unproven uses in homeopathic doses include the treatment of liver and gallbladder problems.

CAUTION: Do not use during pregnancy.

Notes: The shredded bark and roots of both species was simmered in water to make a bright yellow dye.

Wildlife/veterinary uses: Berries are eaten by birds. The Saanich people claim the berries to be an antidote to shellfish poisoning. They chewed *M. aquifolium* for protection after hunting when approached by a dying deer. Oregon grape is an ingredient in a training mix and nervous system formulas for horses.

Buckthorn; Cascara Buckthorn
Rhamnus alnifolia L'Hér.; *R. purshiana* (DC.) Cooper

Description: Bush or small tree 4 to 20 feet in height. Many branched, thornless, densely foliated. When mature, the bark is gray brown with gray-white lenticels. Leaves thin, hairy on the ribs, fully margined, elliptical to ovate, 2 inches in length. Greenish white flowers are numerous and grow on axillary cymes. Flowers are very small, and five petals. The ripe fruit is red, to black purple with two or three seeds. *R. purshiana* (cascara buckthorn) is taller, to 30 feet, with leaves that have twenty to twenty-four veins. White flowers are in clusters.

Location: *R. alnifolia:* dunelands of Lake Michigan and other lake dune areas. *R. purshiana:* foothills of British Columbia, Idaho, Washington, Montana, and Oregon.

Food: Not edible.

Traditional uses: Prior to World War II, you could find cascara tablets over the counter as a laxative in lieu of Ex-Lax or the like. Native Americans used the bark infusion as a purgative, laxative, and worm-killing tea. An infusion of the twigs and fruit in decoction were used as an emetic. Curing the bark for a year is said to reduce its harshness.

Modern uses: The bark extract of *P. purshiana* is a powerful laxative. It is Commission E–approved for treating constipation. The laxative response may last eight hours.

CAUTION: The drug should never be used to clear intestinal obstructions. Bark infusion is considered a cleansing tonic, but chronic, continuous use may be carcinogenic. Use only under the care of a physician, holistic or otherwise.

Notes: A couple of naturopathic physicians once laced my salmon with the bark extract of cascara as a practical joke. Some joke! My experience was far worse than any bout with the "Mexican quick step." Berries from a *Rhamnus* species I test-tasted in the Midwest once ruined an anniversary dinner. These berries can be mistaken for edible fruit with rueful consequences.

Wildlife/veterinary uses: A natural product containing cascara claims to help rebuild damaged nerves in horses. Cascara taken internally by animals may not have the same physiological effect as with humans.

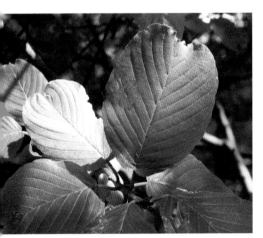

Cascara buckthorn, *Rhamnus purshiana*

American Yew
Taxus brevifolia Nutt.

Description: Evergreen shrub to scanty small tree to 50 feet in height. Bark papery, reddish-purple to red brown. Drooping branches. Flat leaves (needles), in opposite rows. Flowers are small cones. Fruit scarlet, berrylike, with fleshy cup around a single seed.

Location: Northern California, Oregon, and Washington through Idaho and Montana north to British Columbia and Alberta. Foothills; moist, shady sites.

Food: According to Moerman (*Native American Ethnobotany*), the Karok and Mendocino tribes ate the red, ripe fruit. But the seed and all other parts of the plant are toxic. Avoid eating this plant.

Traditional uses: Native Americans used the wet needles of American yew (*T. brevifolia*) as a poultice over wounds. The needles were considered a panacea, a powerful tonic, and were boiled and used over injuries to alleviate pain. Bark decoctions were used to treat stomachache. Native Americans were the first to use this plant to treat cancer.

Modern uses: The toxic drug taxine (paclitaxel) from American yew is used to treat cancer. It prevents cell multiplication and may prove an effective therapy for leukemia and for cancer of the cervix, ovary, and breast. Clinical trials continue with the drug.

CAUTION: Both species can induce abortion. All parts of the plant are toxic. Unless guided by an expert, avoid eating any part of this plant.

Notes: Research reports that the cancer-fighting chemistry is in both species. It takes nearly 3,000 trees or 9,000 kilograms of dried inner bark of *T. brcvifolia* to make 1 kilogram of the drug Taxol. At that rate all of the wild yew trees in America would be destroyed to produce the needed supply of the drug! Taxol today is grown in culture from cloned cells in huge bioreactor tanks, and nary a tree is destroyed. Researchers are attempting to produce the drug from pinene from pine trees.

Wildlife/veterinary uses: Birds and small mammals eat fruit and disperse seed. Moose, deer, and elk browse foliage in winter. Heavy browse in western Montana and northern Idaho has reduced the tree to a shrubby form. Yew snags are habitat for cavity-nesting birds.

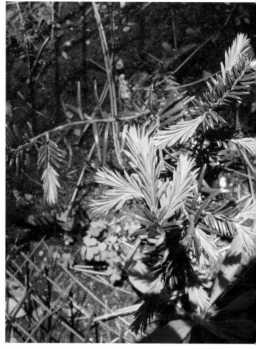

Yews, *Taxus brevifolia*

CHAPTER 8

Medicinal Plants of the Desert

*We told the white man to let us alone, and keep
away from us; but they followed on, and beset our
paths, and they coiled themselves among us, like
the snake. They poisoned us by their touch.*

—CHIEF BLACK HAWK

These medicinal plants are found in arid biomes of the western United States and Mexico.

Sage, Sagebrush

Artemisia tridentata Nutt.

Description: Gray, fragrant shrub to 7 feet. Leaves are wedged shaped, lobed (three teeth) broad at tip, tapering to the base. Yellow and brownish flowers form spreading, long, narrow clusters. Bloom in July to October. Seed is hairy achene.

Location: Dry areas of Wyoming, Washington, Montana, Texas, New Mexico, California, Idaho, Oregon, Colorado . . .

Food: Seeds, raw or dried, are ground into flour and eaten as a survival food. Seeds have been added to liqueurs for fragrance and flavor.

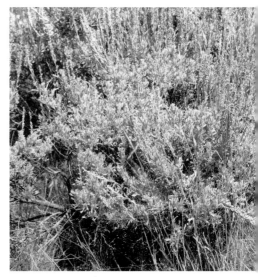

Sage, *Artemisia tridentata*

Traditional uses: This powerful warrior plant is used for smudging and sweeping to rid the victim of bad airs and evil spirits. Leaves are used as a tea to treat infec-tions or ease childbirth or as a wash for sore eyes. Leaves are soaked in water and applied as a poultice over wounds.

The tea is used to treat stomachache. Tree limbs are used as switches in sweat baths. The infusion was used to treat sore throats, coughs, colds, and bronchitis. A decoction or infusion was used as a wash for sores, cuts, and pimples. The aromatic decoction of steaming herb was inhaled for respiratory ailments and headaches. The decoction was said to be internally antidiarreal and externally antirheumatic. This panacea drug was also drunk to relieve constipation.

Modern uses: Still very popular and important in Native American Church rituals, including smudging, sweeping, sweat lodge, and as a disinfectant. For details see the DVD *Native American Medicine* (appendix D).

Notes: Add this herb to your hot bath, hot tub, or sweat lodge for a fragrant, disinfecting, and relaxing cleanse. Often sagebrush is the only source of firewood in the desert.

Wildlife/veterinary uses: Native Americans rubbed the herb over their bodies to hide the human scent when hunting. Considered a moth and flea repellent, the decoction of the herb was applied to the wounds of domestic animals.

Prickly Pear
Opuntia spp.

Description: Desert cactus with oval pads and thorny leaves of various sizes. Flowers yellowish. Fruits variable, typically white to red to purple.

Location: Various species found from coast to coast in dry, sometimes sandy areas.

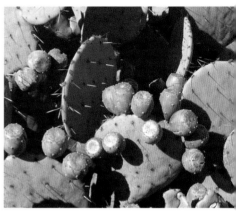
Prickly pear, *Opuntia* sp.

Food: The pads, which are often mistaken for leaves (actually the spines are the leaves), are edible. Most edible species have flat joints between pads. Flowers and flower buds are roasted and eaten. Species with plump pads (the new growth is preferred) may be thrown on hot coals of fire and roasted. The fire burns off the spines and cooks the interior. Let the pads cool, then peel the skin and eat the inner core. I like to slice the inner "meat" and stir-fry it, or I chop the pad "meat" into huevos rancheros with yucca blossoms and salsa verde. I have eaten the flowers of several species, as have Native American foragers, but there is little about this practice in the literature. Do so at your own risk. The fruit when red and ripe is tasty and often made into jelly. I like to eat it out of hand right off plant (avoid the prickly hairs). The pads can be mixed with water, sugar, yeast and fermented into an alcoholic drink. The young green fruit is boiled and eaten by Pima Indians.

Traditional uses: The flowers are astringent and can be poulticed over wounds.

Flowers prepared as a tea are taken for stomach complaints including diarrhea and irritable bowel syndrome. The stem ash is applied to burns and cuts. Pima Indians believed the edible pads are good for gastrointestinal complaints. Leaf pads are scorched of spines, then sliced in half and the moist side applied as a poultice for cleansing and sealing wounds, infections, bites, stings, and snake envenomations. The Pimas despined, cooked, sliced, and poulticed plants on breasts as a lactagogue. The infusion of stems of a Sonoran desert species, *O. polyacantha* (plains prickly pear), was used to treat diarrhea.

Modern uses: In Mexico and the American Southwest, prickly pear is used in its traditional ways. According to Andrew Chevallier (*Encyclopedia of Medicinal Plants*), the flowers are still used for treating an enlarged prostate.

Notes: The inner flesh of the pad is a chemotactic attractant, a surfactant, that draws serum from the wound site, thus cleaning and sealing it. Try the fruit peeled, sliced, and eaten with a spicy dose of cayenne pepper.

Wildlife/veterinary uses: *Opuntia* pads are sliced open and applied, moist side down, over wounds, bites, stings, and envenomations. Southwestern holistic practitioners report success in treating scorpion and recluse spider bites. I suspect the gel applied to an animal's wounds would be just as effective as it is with humans. Because of this thorny plant's aggressive, invasive nature, it is problematic to grazing animals. But goats will eat it as starvation food. I have seen

antelope graze on flowers, and in a pinch they will eat the pads.

Yucca: Adam's Needle; Spanish Bayonet; Joshua Tree

Yucca spp.: *Y. filamentosa* L.; *Y. glauca* Nutt.; *Y. baccata* Torr.

Description: Perennials with large, ever-expanding rootstocks, often growing in clumps and colonies. Leaves swordlike, radiating out from basal rosettes, waxy (shiny) green; long, tough and fibrous. Flowers white or cream colored; cup, bell, or bowl shaped; borne on tall woody spikes extending well above leaves. Typically flowers from May through July.

Location: Upland prairies, plains, sandy blowouts, hillsides.

Food: We eat the white flowers from this plant. Fold them fresh into frittatas or omelets. Garnish a plate with them. Shred them onto salads. The fruits of these plants are also edible, a few species more edible than others. *Y. baccata* has large succulent fruits that are

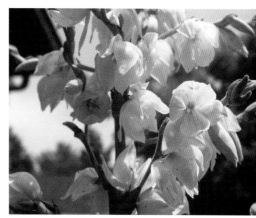

Yucca, *Yucca glauca*

bland but rich with health-protecting flavonoids.

Traditional uses: Folklore claims that the root decoction will restore hair. The infusion of the smashed root was taken internally to relieve headache. Yucca root extract is a surfactant or wetting agent, capable of popping the cell membranes of microorganisms. It is therefore a useful, natural soap. Yucca root water decoction is still used to wash hair and kill lice. The root water decoction was drunk to treat arthritis (phytosterols), a potentially risky proposition with so little scientific study of the plant having been performed. See the video *Little Medicine: The Wisdom to Avoid Big Medicine* (appendix D). *Y. filamentosa* root, with its steroid saponins, has been decocted and used to treat gallbladder and liver problems. A water extraction of smashed leaves was used to quell vomiting, and root water infusion used as a laxative. The root is a male warrior plant and used in smudging rituals to rid the body of bad airs and bad spirits. The root of *Y. baccata* was taken to ease childbirth; this author surmises that the bitter saponins stimulated contractions.

Modern uses: In Europe leaves ground and dried and extracts of the plant are available for medicinal use. The root and leaf extraction (steroid saponins) of Adam's needle, *Y. filamentosa,* are still used for liver and gallbladder complaints. The side effects of too much steroid saponin intake are stomach upset and nausea. These uses are scientifically unconfirmed.

Notes: Yucca flower shoots—the tall stalks that bear the flowers—are dried and used by Native Americans as arrow shafts and fire-starting spindles for Indian matches. See the video *Survival: Seventeen Ways to Start a Fire Without a Match* (www.herbvideos.com). Yucca plants will grow in your yard or garden and are fun to have around.

Veterinarian/wildlife: One cubic inch of the roots of *Y. baccata* or *Y. filamatosa* may be pureed in 2 cups of water, strained, and filtered into a plant spray. Add another pint of water and use this insecticidal spray on fruit and vegetables. It's organic, water soluble, and a good alternative to more toxic sprays. Early informants suggested that Native Americans pounded yucca roots into water to stun fish. Experiments I have conducted suggest it is the aerial part of the plant, principally the leaves, that knock out fish. The root water actually appeared to stimulate my little finned friends. Yucca extracts are used in lawn-guard formulations that protect your yard from the brown die-off caused by pets urinating on the grass. Various horse supplement contain yucca, including joint support formulations and hoof and foot support supplements.

Agave, American Century Plant

Agave spp.: *A. americana* L.

Description: Grayish green desert plant to 10 feet. Long, swordlike, succulent leaves.

Location: Extreme southwestern United States—California, Arizona, Nevada, and Mexico; Central and South America.

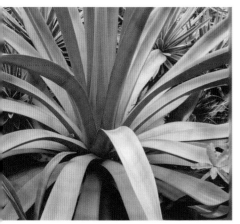

Agave, *Agave americana*

Food: American century plant roots are pit cooked, crushed in water, and fermented. Young leaves are roasted and eaten or stored for later use. Fruit heads, young buds, and flower stalks are roasted and eaten (I have also eaten the flowers). Agave is made into pulque, vino mescal, and tequila. Mescal agave "leaves" are cut out from center of plant, then "water" from the plant weeps into the hole. A pulque farmer, using a hollow calabash with a cow horn snout fused to one end, sucks watery sap into gourd. The sap is fermented in buckets for six or seven days, then served. Agave water harvested in this way is used as potable drinking water. Every Hispanic worth his or her salt (and a squirt of lime) grows an agave. Demand for tequila has greatly inflated the plant's value. Disease is also threatening the crop, and urban sprawl in Mexico leaves less land available for cultivation. The core of the tender inner leaves of the plant may be cooked and eaten.

Traditional uses: Agave water (juice, sap) is considered anti-inflammatory and diuretic. Also the fresh juice may raise metabolism and increase perspiration.

Modern uses: Leaf waste is gathered, concentrated, and used as starter material for steroid drugs (hecogenin). Agave roots contain suds-producing saponins and are used in the manufacture of soap products. The coarse fiber from leaves is used to make rope and fiber (sisal is manufactured from *A. sisalana*). The sap continues to be used as a demulcent and laxative.

Notes: The sap is used for treating and sealing wounds. Cortez dropped his ax half through his thigh and surely would have died had not the Mesoamerican natives stopped the bleeding and sealed the wound with a compress of sticky agave leaf sap, honey, and charcoal.

Wildlife/veterinary uses: The root extraction is an insecticide. Seed production from an agave plant drops without bats as pollinators. *A. lecheguilla* has caused hepatotoxicosis in grazing animals, characterized by an itching photodermatitis and swelling of the skin.

Gumweed

Grindelia camporum Green; *G. integrifolia* DC.; *G. nana* Nutt.

Description: All species are similar; *G. camporum* is described here: Erect biennial or perennial to 3½ feet in height but typically smaller. Light green leaves are alternate, ovate to oblong, serrated or smooth margins, with a clasping the stem, often resin dotted. Flowers yellow to yellow orange, dandelion-like (composite). Flower bracts are viscous and sticky, hence the name gumweed.

Location: *G. camporum:* Southwestern United States to California, up the Sonoran desert to British Columbia and other dry areas of the West. *G. integrifolia* is a Northwest coastal plant of salt marshes and open coastlines. *G. nana* is found in Idaho.

Food: Not edible.

Traditional uses: Used to treat upper respiratory infections. Native Americans used the plant decoction externally to treat wounds, poison ivy and poison oak, boils, and unspecified dermatitis. Sticky leaves and flowers were applied to the sores.

Modern uses: Commission E–approved for treating bronchitis and cough. The resinous drug has shown in vitro studies to be antimicrobial, antifungal, and anti-inflammatory. Dried aerial parts are used in tea or tincture.

CAUTION: Large doses may be poisonous and a gastric irritant.

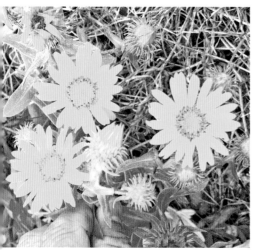

Gumweed, *Grindelia integrifolia*

Notes: A variety of species are seen as one travels the backroads diagonally across the upper West from Yellowstone to Vancouver. Gumweed is primarily found in dry areas, but you'll see the marine variety, *G. integrifolia,* when you reach the Pacific coast.

Wildlife/veterinary uses: Flathead First Peoples rubbed curlycup gumweed (*G. squarrosa*) flower heads on horses' hooves for protection against injury. A decoction of tops and leaves of an unspecified gumweed was used as a wash for saddle galls and sores on horses.

Morman Tea, Joint Fir; Ephedra, Ma Huang
Ephedra viridis Coville; *E. sinica*

Description: There are several joint fir species. *E. viridis* looks like it has lost all its leaves. It is a yellow green plant, many jointed and twiggy, 1 to 4 feet tall, with small leaf scales, and double seeded cones in the fall.

Location: Various species are found on dry rocky soil or sand in desertlike areas of the United States: Utah, Arizona, western New Mexico, Colorado, Nevada, California, Oregon.

Food: Native Americans infused the roasted seeds. Roasted and ground seeds were mixed with corn or wheat flour to make fried mush.

Traditional uses: *E. viridis*, Mormon tea, was used in infusion as a tonic and laxative; to treat anemia, colds, ulcers, and backache; to stem diarrhea; and as therapy for the kidneys and bladder. The

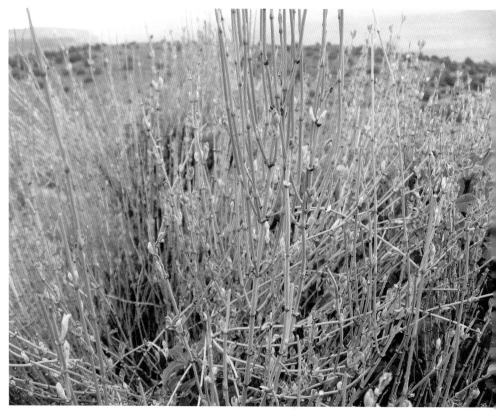

Mormon tea, *Ephedra viridis*

decoction or infusion is considered a cleansing tonic (blood purifier). Dried and powdered stems were used externally to treat wounds and sores. The powder was also moistened and applied to burns. It was used by First Peoples to stimulate delayed mentrual flow (dysmenorrhea). Seeds were roasted before being brewed into tea.

Modern uses: The Chinese species *E. sinica* is commonly used today. In China the dried jointed stems are powdered and used to treat coughs and bronchitis, bronchial asthma, congestion, hay fever, and obesity (as a stimulant). It's also used as an appetite suppressant and basal metabolism stimulant. American ephedra is available as a tea or in capsules over the counter and has little or no vasoactive effects, unlike *E. sinica*.

CAUTION: *E. sinica*, as a cardiovascular stimulant and central nervous system stimulant, may be dangerous to people with elevated blood pressure, heart disease, or tachycardia. It is federally regulated and is not to be used during pregnancy or by nursing mothers. Numerous drug interactions have been documented. The import and use of this drug is restricted in several countries. Deaths have been associated with its abuse.

Notes: I have enjoyed the twig tea of the American variety while filming wild plants in the Four Corners area around Mesa Verde.

Wildlife/veterinary uses: The twigs can be dried and powdered, carried in your first-aid kit, and applied to cuts, scraps, wounds, stings, and bites—on you, your dog, or your horse. If available, cover the powdered ephedra with a slice of prickly pear pad.

Jojoba
Simmondsia chinensis (Link) Schneid.

Description: Evergreen shrub with many branches and separate sexed plants (dioecious). Thick blue green leaves, oblong and paired. Male flowers small, yellow in color. Female flower has small inconspicuous pale green flowers. Fruit capsule has one to three seeds, with single-seeded most common.

Location: Sonora desert, desert Southwest, and into Mexico. Cultivated in the Southwest for liquid wax.

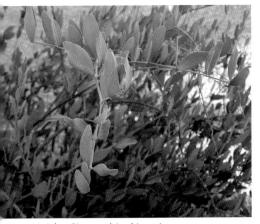

Jojoba, *Simmondsia chinensis*

Food: Seeds are ground and percolated or decocted into a coffeelike drink. Waxy seed kernels are boiled or baked and eaten or blended into cake mix. Nuts can be shelled and eaten. Parched nut kernels are made into nut butter.

Traditional uses: Native Americans of the Southwest dried the nuts, pulverized them, and applied the mass to wounds and sores. The nutlike fruit was powdered and taken internally for catharsis, but it was used primarily as a dermatological to treat acne and psoriasis. Chewing raw, green jojoba seeds was a treatment for sore throats.

Modern uses: Used as carrier oil for skin care products, the seed extract protects principal ingredients from oxidation. Jojoba has possible cholesterol-lowering potential, but more studies are needed.

Notes: Widely cultivated in the Southwest and used for skin health. No contraindications exist when the product is used as prescribed on the package.

Wildlife/veterinary uses: Jojoba shampoo may be used on pets and horses to soothe skin and scalp conditions.

Chaparral, Creosote Bush
Larrea tridentata (Sessé & Moc. ex DC.) Coville

Description: Resinous and aromatic shrub to 6 feet. Reddish brown bark near the base, lighter to almost white higher up and on limbs and branches. Leaves small, yellow green, with glossy leathery look and texture. Flowers tiny, yellow colored, developing into fuzzy (hairy) seed-bearing capsules.

Location: Southwestern United States and Mexico. Desert.

Food: Toxic, not edible.

Traditional uses: A decoction of the evergreen leaves of the creosote bush was used by various North American Indian tribes to treat diarrhea and stomach problems. A poultice of the chewed plant was placed over insect bites, spider bites, and snakebites. A wash of leaf infusion was used to increase milk flow. Sap from heated twigs was packed into cavities to treat toothache, and a leaf poultice was applied to wounds and skin problems and as a therapy for chest complaints. Documented Native American uses included chaparral as a treatment for rheumatic disease, venereal infections, urinary infections, and cancer, especially leukemia. A tea made from the leaves was taken internally as an expectorant and pulmonary antiseptic.

Modern uses: Until recently chaparral was widely used to treat many conditions, including fever, influenza, colds, gas, arthritis, sinusitis, anemia, fungal infections, allergies, autoimmunity diseases, and premenstrual syndrome. It is considered an analgesic, antidiarrheal, diuretic, and emetic. The leaves and small twigs were collected, washed, and dried and then ground into an oily powder yeilding the drug.

CAUTION: Today the commercial and medical use of chaparral is suspect due to concern over its potential toxic effect upon the liver, causing subacute or acute hepatitis. The chemistry of chaparral is well studied, and extensive literature has been published on the principal lignan

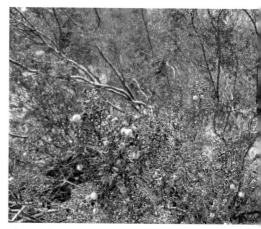

Chaparral, *Larrea tridentata*

component, NDGA (nordihydroguaiaretic acid). NDGA is a powerful antioxidant—in animal studies it has shown to be both anticancer and cancer promoting. Because of the cancer-causing potential, the questions concerning liver toxicity, and the unproven uses of the herb, it is best to consider an alternative to chaparral. In 2005 Health Canada warned consumers not to ingest the herb chaparral in the form of loose leaves, teas, capsules, or bulk herbal products because of the risk of liver and kidney problems. Holistic health-care professionals may still recommend and use the herb, but it is this author's contention that use of chaparral should be avoided until evidence of efficacy and safety are scientifically established.

Notes: One of the reasons for the chaparral's great success is the presence a highly toxic substance produced in and released from its root that prevents other plants from growing nearby. Rainfall washes away the toxin, allowing other plants to grow. Once the water drains off, the toxin is released again and the invading plants are destroyed. This ability ensures that chaparral does not have to compete with other plant life for scarce desert nutrients.

Wildlife/veterinary uses: Used as an insecticide and fish poison. Twigs were made into war and hunting arrow shafts.

Yaupon, Yaupon Holly
Ilex vomitoria Ait.

Description: Evergreen holly, shrublike. Hollylike leaves are oval, alternating, glossy green; margins lined with round teeth.

Location: Texas and throughout the Southwest and southeastern states as far north as North Carolina. A borderline desert plant.

Food: Berries are toxic, but the leaves can be roasted into tea. Gather a mix of young leaves from near the tips and old leaves from the branch. Roast leaves at 200°F until the green turns brown. Put a crushed teaspoon of leaves in a cup of water and microwave on high for ninety seconds. Cool and drink.

Traditional uses: Leaves and fruit were used in ritual healing by numerous First People nations. A decoction of the roasted leaves was used to purge organ systems and as an emetic. Sipping the decoction helped older people sleep by quelling nightmares. It is said to cure talking in sleep and restlessness. It is considered hallucinogenic.

Modern uses: Leaves are roasted then steeped in water to make a light tea as a

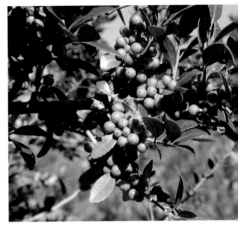

Yaupon, *Ilex vomitoria*

diuretic and stimulant. Strong infusions are used in purification rituals to purify the body through vomiting. The stimulating property comes form the presence of caffeine in the plant, much like the beverage Mate infused from the South American holly, *I. paraquariensis*.

CAUTION: The berries are toxic.

Notes: The long, straight branches were used to make ramrods for flintlock guns and arrow shafts. The leaves and berries can be used to make dyes. The ripe red berries make a red dye in a mordant of alum water. Use the dye on wool: Place the wool item in the dye and let the color infuse in full sunlight. Grays can be achieved by mixing leaves in water with iron and or copper.

Wildlife/veterinary uses: This plant is an excellent addition to the homestead garden to attract cedar waxwings, robins, mockingbirds, and brown thrashers.

Appendix A:
Longevity Index

When you consider that the United States has the costliest and reportedly best health-care system in the world, then the following statistics make you wonder. Here are a few countries that are getting it right and whose citizens are zealous foragers of wild edibles.

Life expectancy in years:

New Zealand: 81.1
Japan: 81.0
Greece: 78.9
Italy: 78.7
United States: 77.2

Appendix B: Jim Meuninck's Top Eleven Garden Herbs

1. Garlic: infection fighter, stimulant
2. Rosemary: cancer-fighting antioxidants, stimulant
3. Basil: antioxidants, infection fighter
4. Mint: stimulant, digestive
5. Lemon balm: relaxing tonic for mild depression, irritability, anxiety
6. Fennel: anti-inflammatory, analgesic, appetite stimulant, antiflatulent
7. Lovage: respiratory and digestive tonic, antibronchitic
8. Oregano: antiseptic, antiflatulent, stimulate bile and stomach acid, antiasthmatic
9. Cilantro (coriander): to treat flatulence, bloating and cramps; breath sweetener
10. Horseradish: perspirant, stimulant
11. Thyme: tea for preventing altitude sickness, antiseptic, inhalant (antiasthmatic), stimulant

Appendix C:
Helpful Web Sites

http://nccam.nih.gov. U.S. Office of Alternative and Complementary Medicine
www.ars-grin.gov/duke. Database of medicinal plant chemistry
www.cinim.org. Canadian Institute of Natural and Integrative Medicine
www.clinicaltrials.gov. Online source of clinical trials in the United States
www.ethnobotany.com. How people use plants as medicine
www.herbalgram.org. American Botanical Council
www.herbvideos.com. Jim Meuninck's site, thousand of pages with photos and links
www.rain-tree.com. Amazon rain forest plants and their medicinal uses

Appendix D:
References and Resources

Aller, Wilma. "Aboriginal Food Utilization of Vegetation by Indians of the Great Lakes Region as Recorded in the Jesuit Relations." *Wisconsin Archaeologist* (1954): 59–73.

Atkinson, Charlotte, Juliet E. Compston, Nicholas E. Day, et al. "The Effects of Phytoestrogen Isoflavones on Bone Density in Women: A Double-blind Randomized, Placebo-Controlled Trial." *American Journal of Clinical Nutrition* 79, no. 2 (2004): 326–33.

Barrett, S. A. "The Washoe Indians." *Bulletin of the Public Museum of Milwaukee* (1917).

Basehart, Harry. *Mescalero Apache Subsistence Patterns and Socio-Political Organization.* Garland Publishing, 1974.

Blumenthal, Mark, ed., et al. *The Complete German Commission E Monographs: Therapeutic Guide to Herbal Medicines.* American Botanical Council; Integrative Medicine Communications, 1998.

Blumenthal, Mark, Alicia Goldberg, and Joseph Brinckmann, eds. *Herbal Medicine: Expanded Commission E Monographs.* American Botanical Council; Integrative Medicine Communications, 1999.

Bradley, Will. "Medical Practices of New England Aborigines." *Journal of the American Pharmaceutical Association* (1936): 138.

Brill, Steve, and Evelyn Dean. *Identifying and Harvesting Edible and Medicinal Plants in Wild (and Not So Wild) Places.* Hearst Books, 1994.

Brown, Deni. *Encyclopedia of Herbs and Their Uses.* Dorling Kindersley, 1995.

Campbell, T. "Medicinal Plants of the Choctaw, Chickasaw, and Creek Indians in the Early Nineteenth Century." *Journal of the Washington Academy of Sciences* (1951): 285–90.

Carr, L., and C. Westey. "Surviving Folktales and Herbal Lore among the Shinnecock Indians." *Journal of American Folklore* (1945): 113–23.

Chevallier, Andrew. *Encyclopedia of Medicinal Plants.* Reader's Digest Association, 1996.

Color Atlas of Chinese Traditional Drugs. National Institute for the Control of Pharmaceutical and Biological Products; Science Press, Beijing, China, 1987.

Coville, Frederick. "Notes on the Plants Used by the Klamath Indians of Oregon." Contributions from the U.S. National Herbarium (1897): 87–110.

Duke, James. *Biological Active Phytochemicals and Their Activities*. CRC Press, 1992.

———. *Handbook of Edible Weeds*. CRC Press, 2001.

———. *Handbook of Medicinal Herbs*. CRC Press, 2001.

———. *Handbook of Northeastern Indian Medicinal Plants*. Quarterman Publications, 1986.

———. *Phytochemical Constituents of GRAS Herbs and Other Economic Plants*. CRC Press, 1992.

Fava, M., et al. "A Double-blind, Randomized Trial of St. John's Wort, Fluoxetine, and Placebo in Major Depressive Disorder." *Journal of Clinical Psychopharmocology* 25, no. 5 (2005): 441–47.

Fewkes, Walter. "A Contribution to Ethnobotany." *American Anthropologist* 9 (1896): 14–21.

Fletcher, Alice, and Francis Flesche. "The Omaha Tribe." *Smithsonian Institution Bureau of Ethnology Annual Report,* no. 27 (1911).

Foster, Steven, and James A. Duke. *A Field Guide to Medicinal Plants: Eastern and Central North America*. Houghton Mifflin, 1990.

Gilmore, Melvin. *Some Chippewa Uses of Plants*. University of Michigan Press, 1933.

———. *A Study in the Ethnobotany of the Omaha Indians*. Nebraska State Historical Society Collections 17 (1913): 314–57.

———. *Uses of Plants by the Indians of the Missouri River Region*. University of Nebraska Press, 1914, 1991.

Gunter, Erna. *Ethnobotany of Western Washington.* University of Washington Press, 1944, 1995.

Harrington, John. "Tobacco among the Karuk Indians of California." *Smithsonian Institution Bureau of American Ethnology Bulletin,* no. 91 (1932).

Hart, Jeff. *Montana Native Plants and Early Peoples*. Helena (Montana) Historical Society Press, 1992.

Hsu, Hong-yen, et al. *Oriental Materia Medica: A Concise Guide*. Keats Publishing; Oriental Healing Arts Institute, 1996.

Kapoor, L. D. *Handbook of Ayurvedic Medicinal Plants*. CRC Press, 2001.

Króliczewska, Bozena, and Wojciech Zawadzki. "The Influence of Skullcap Root Addition (*Scutellaria baicalensis radix*) on Calcium, Inorganic Phosphorus, Magnesium, and Iron Levels in Broiler Chicken Serum." Agricultural University of Wrocaw, Poland.

Kucera, M., et al. "Effects of Symphytumn Ointment on Muscular Symptoms and Functional Locomotor Disturbances." *Advanced Therapies* 17, no. 4 (2000): 204–10.

Kuhnlein, Harriet V., and Nancy J. Turner. *Traditional Plant Foods of Canadian Indigenous People.* Gordon and Breach, 1991.

Mandelbaum, David. "The Plains Cree." *Anthropological Papers of the American Museum of Natural History* 37 (1940): 202–03.

Meuninck, Jim. *Basic Essentials Edible Wild Plants,* Falcon, 2006**.**

———. *Herbal Odyssey* (CD). www.herbvideos.com, 2007.

Meuninck, Jim, James Balch, Ed Smith, et al. *Natural Health with Medicinal Herbs and Healing Foods* (DVD). www.herbvideos.com, 2007.

Meuninck, Jim, and Theresa Barnes. *Little Medicine: The Wisdom to Avoid Big Medicine* (DVD). www.herbvideos.com, 2005.

Meuninck, Jim, Patsy Clark, and Theresa Barnes. *Native American Medicine* (DVD). www.herbvideos.com, 2007.

Meuninck, Jim, Candace Corson, and Nancy Behnke Strasser. *Diet for Natural Health: One Diet for Disease Prevention and Weight Control.* www.herbvideos.com, 1999 (video), 2007 (DVD).

Meuninck, Jim, and James Duke. *Edible Wild Plants* (DVD). www.herbvideos.com, 2007.

———. *Trees, Shrubs, Nuts and Berries* (DVD). www.herbvideos.com, 2007.

Meuninck, Jim, and Sinclair Philip. *Cooking with Edible Flowers and Culinary Herbs* (DVD). www.herbvideos.com, 2007.

Moore, Michael. *Medicinal Plants of the Pacific West.* Red Crane Books, 1993.

———. *Medicinal Plants of the Mountain West.* Museum of New Mexico Press, 2003.

Moerman, Daniel. *Native American Ethnobotany.* Timber Press, 1998.

Naegele, Thomas A. *Edible and Medicinal Plants of the Great Lakes Region.* Wilderness Adventure Books, 1996.

Nestel, Pomeroy, Kay, et al. "Isoflavones from Red Clover Improves Systemic Arterial Compliance but Not Plasma Lipids in Menopausal Women." *Journal of Clinical Endocrinological Metabolism* 84, no. 3 (1999): 895–98.

Palmer, Arthur. "Shuswap Indian Ethnobotany." *Syesis* 8 (1975): 29–51.

PDR for Herbal Medicines, third edition. Medical Economics, 2005.

Pojar, Jim, and Andy MacKinnon. *Plants of Coastal British Columbia.* Lone Pine, 1994.

Radhamani, T. R., L. Sudarshana, and R. Krishnan. "Defence and Carnivory: Dual Roles of Bracts in *Passiflora foetida." Journal of Biosciences* 20 (1995): 657–64.

Reid, Daniel. *Chinese Herbal Medicine.* Shambhala, 1987.

Review of Natural Products, fourth edition. Facts and Comparisons, 2005.

Smith, Harlan. "Materia Medica of the Bella Coola and Neighboring Tribe of British Columbia." *National Museum of Canada Bulletin* 56 (1929): 47–68.

Tull, Delena. *Edible and Useful Plants of Texas and the Southwest.* University of Texas Press, 1999.

Van de Weijeer, Barentsen. "Isoflavones from Red Clover (Promensil) Significantly Reduce Menopausal Hot Flush Symptoms Compared with Placebo." *Maturitas* 42, no. 3 (2002): 187–93.

Vestal, Paul. *Ethnobotany of the Ramah Navaho.* Papers of the Peabody Museum of American Archaeology and Ethnology, Harvard University, vol. 40, no. 4., 1952.

Vestal, Paul, and Richard Schultes. *The Economic Botany of the Kiowa Indians.* Botanical Museum, Cambridge, 1939. Reprint, AMS Press, 1981.

Vogel, Virgil. *American Indian Medicine.* University of Oklahoma Press, 1970.

Whitney, Stephen. *Western Forests.* National Audubon Society Nature Guides. Knopf, 1985.

Yanovsky, Elias. *Food Plants of the North American Indians.* USDA Publication 237 (July 1936).

Zicari, D., et al. "Diabetic Retinopathy Treated with Arnica 5 CH Microdoses." *Investigative Ophthalmology & Visual Science* 39 (1998): 118.

Index of Plant Names

Abbreviated Latin names are in parentheses.

About the Author

For forty years biologist Jim Meuninck has traveled the back roads and backwoods of North America, interviewing Native Americans, herbalists, and holistic health-care practitioners to document how Americans use plants as food and medicine. From his research he has authored three books, two CD ROMS, three DVDs, and six videos on the subject. His Web site (www.herbvideos.com) holds more than 3,500 pages of information. He resides on Eagle Lake, Michigan, with his wife, Jill, a Spanish teacher, and his daughter, Rebecca, a graduate student at Michigan State University.

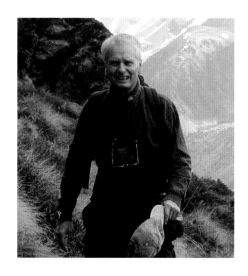

Mike Castleman describes Meuninck in *The Herb Companion* as "a leader in herbal video. His approach to the natural world not only educates, but provides access; he knows what to look for and is out in the field rounding it up for immediate delivery." Steven Foster's *Botanical and Herb Reviews* says: "Meuninck explores what works from Native American traditions in diet and disease prevention. . . . With simple solutions to problems experienced by everyone, his programs are entertaining, informative, and humorous, adding a new dimension to the vast information resources in health."

For information about Jim Meuninck's books and programs, visit his Web site, www.herbvideos.com.

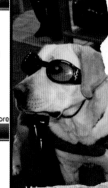
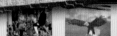